Viruses and Viral Infections in Developing Countries

Edited by Snežana Jovanović-Ćupić, Muhammad Abubakar, Ayşe Emel Önal, Muhammad Kashif Saleemi, Ana Božović and Milena Krajnovic

Published in London, United Kingdom

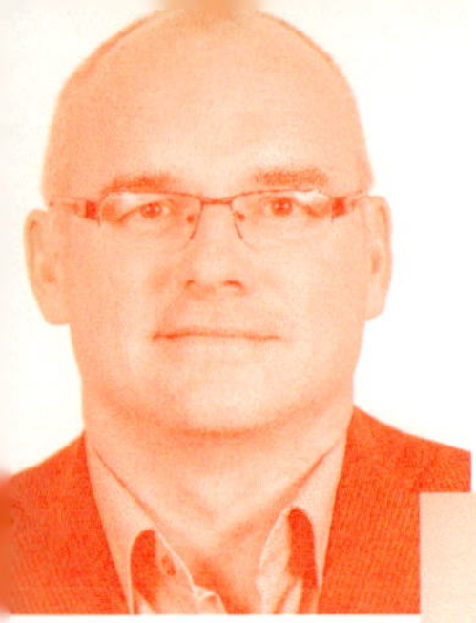
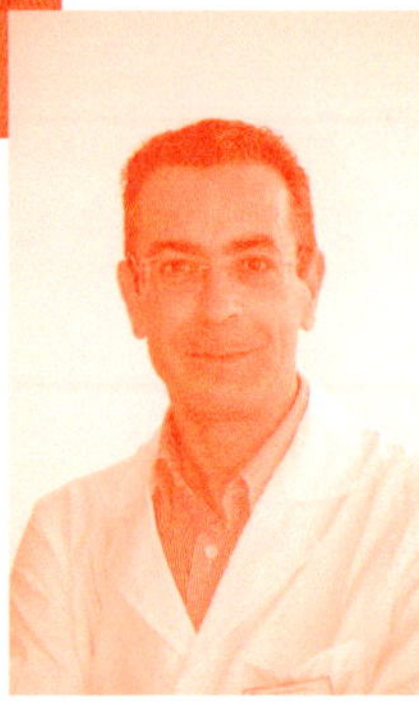
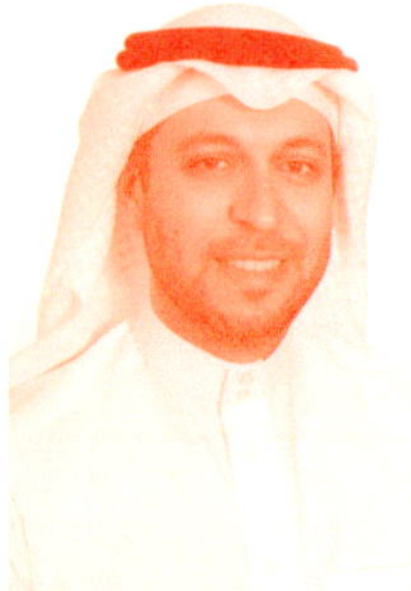
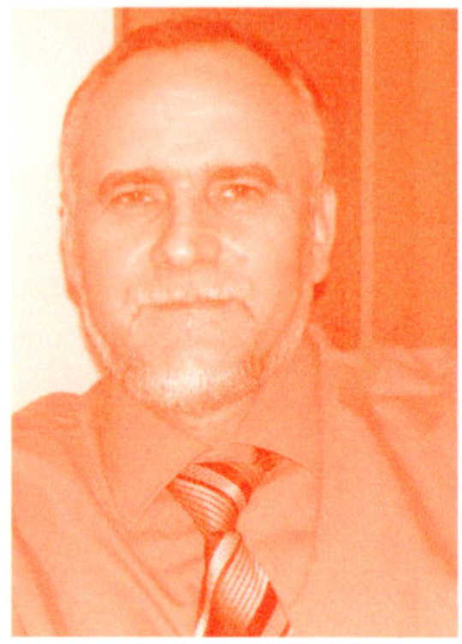
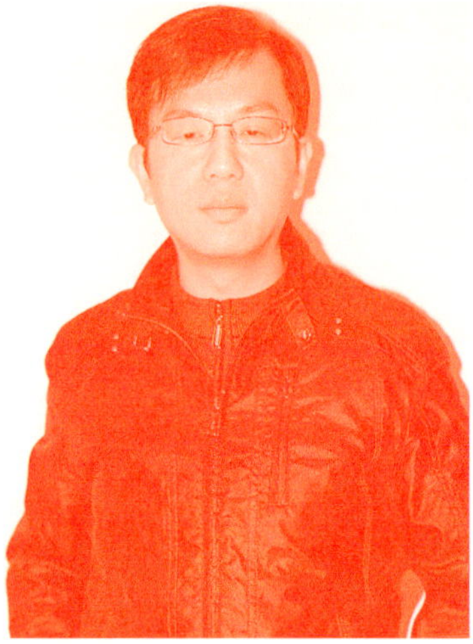
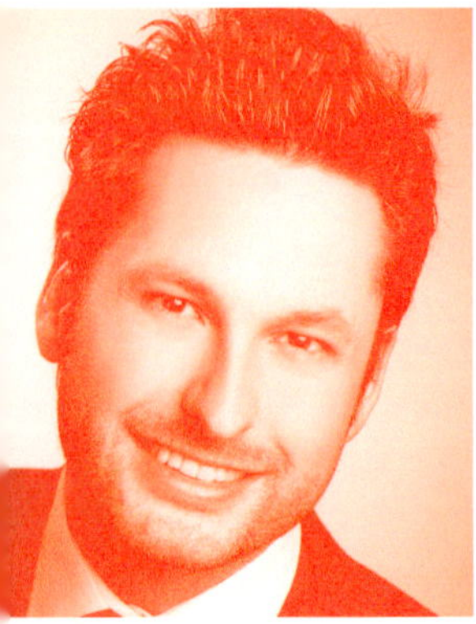
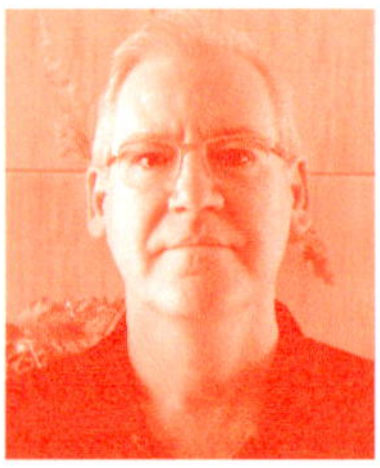

IntechOpen

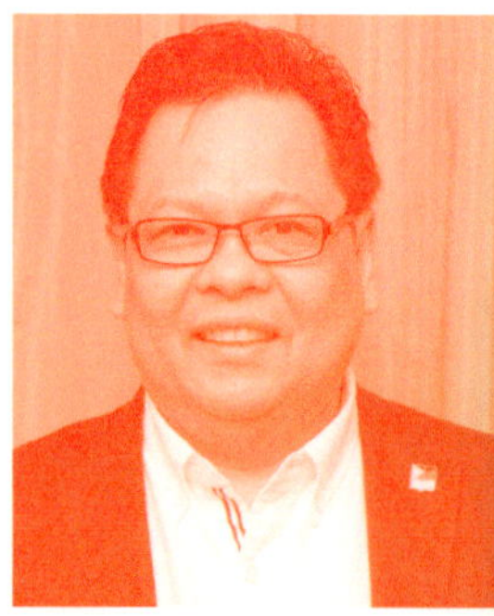
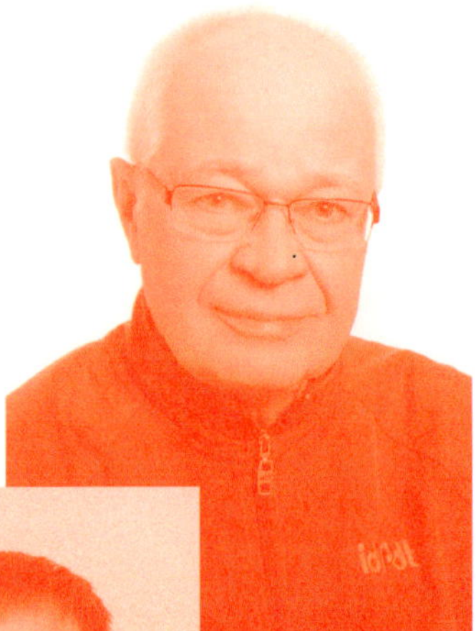
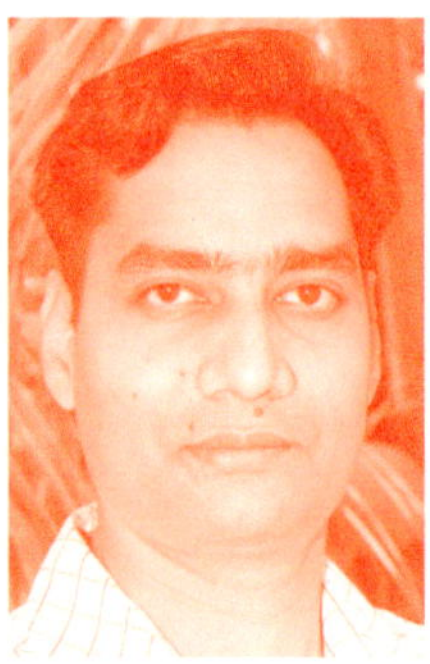
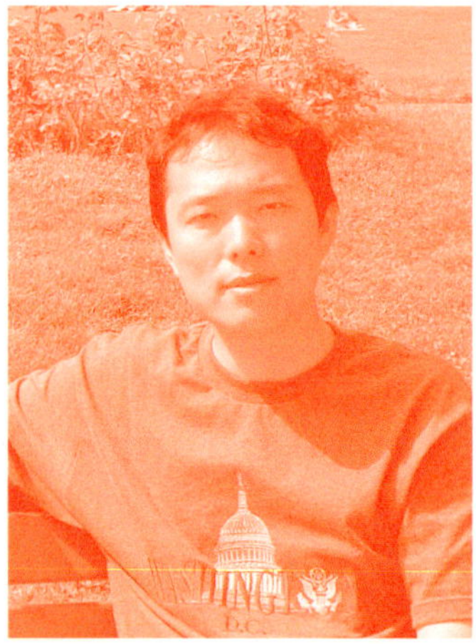
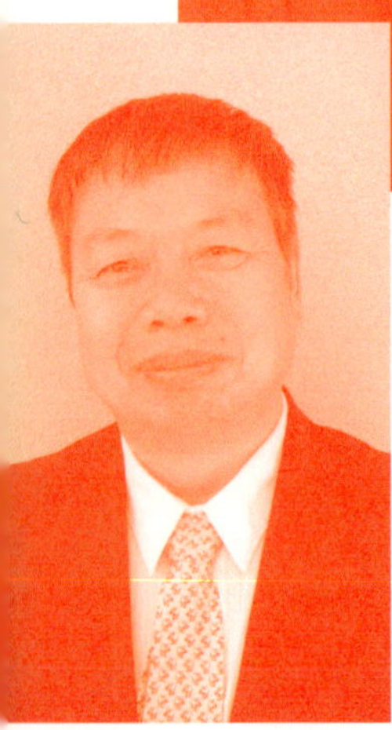
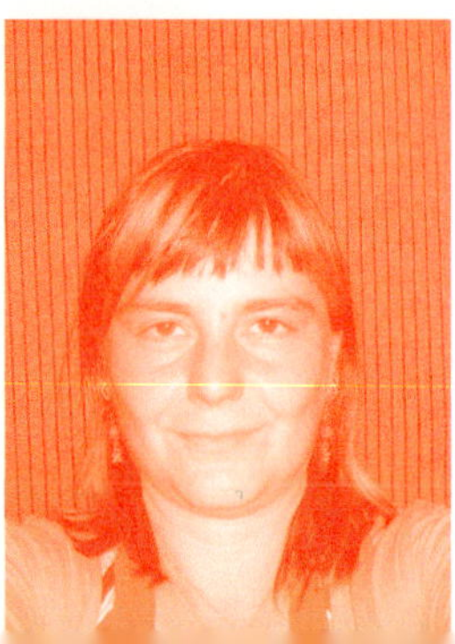

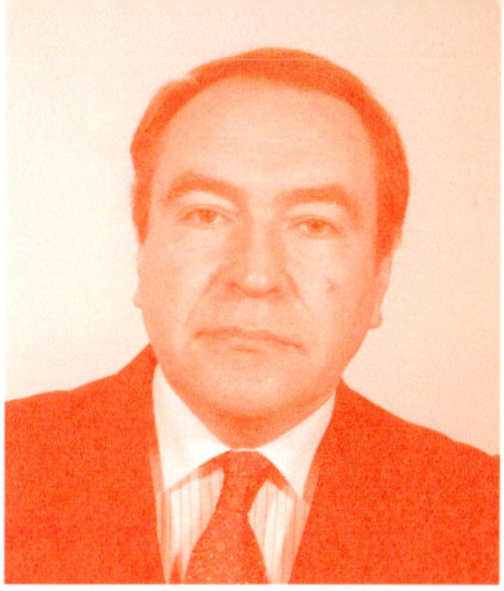
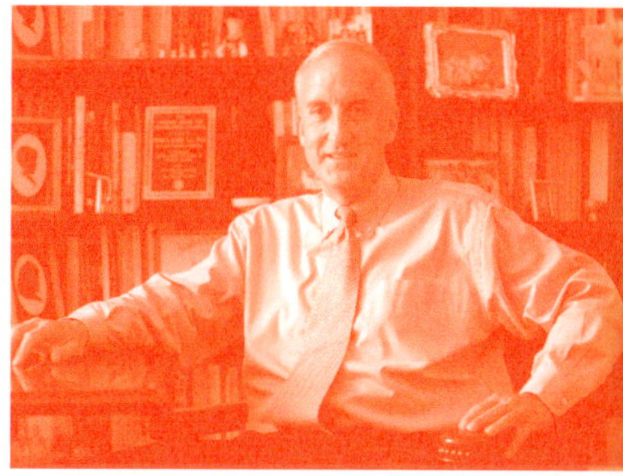
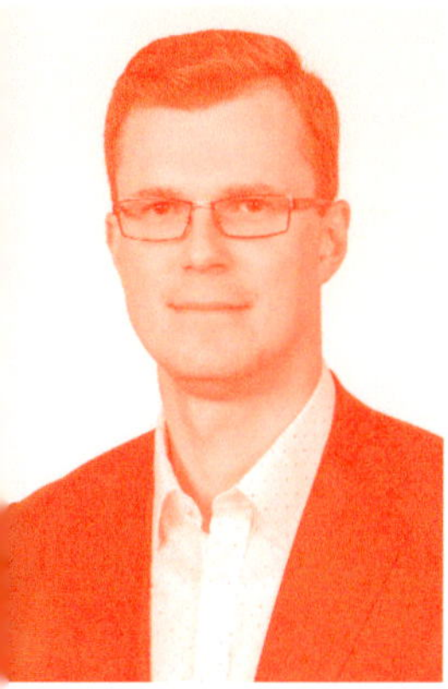
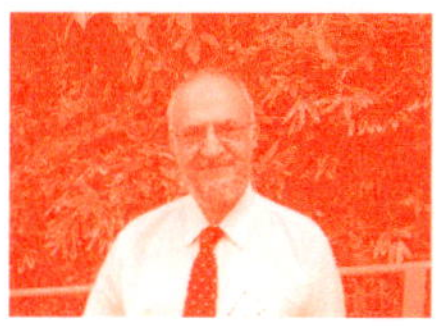
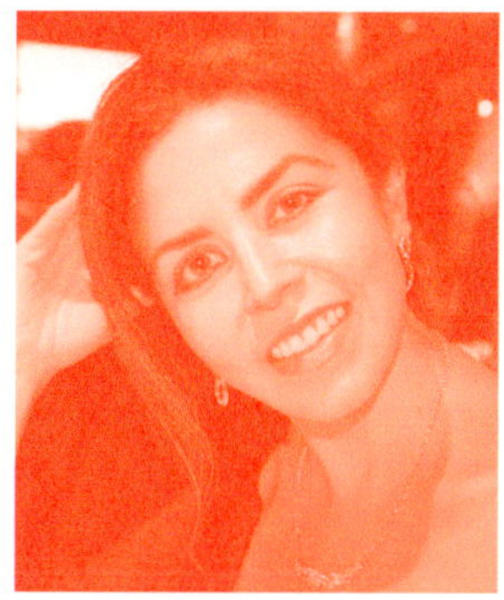

Supporting open minds since 2005

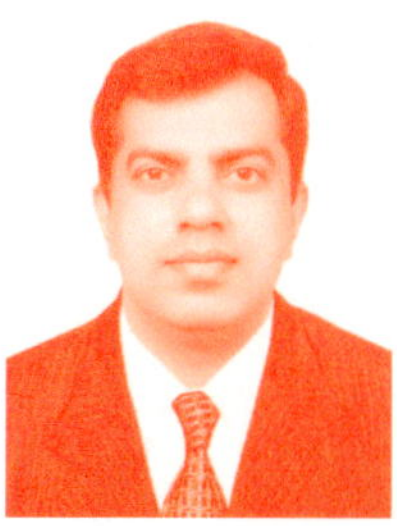
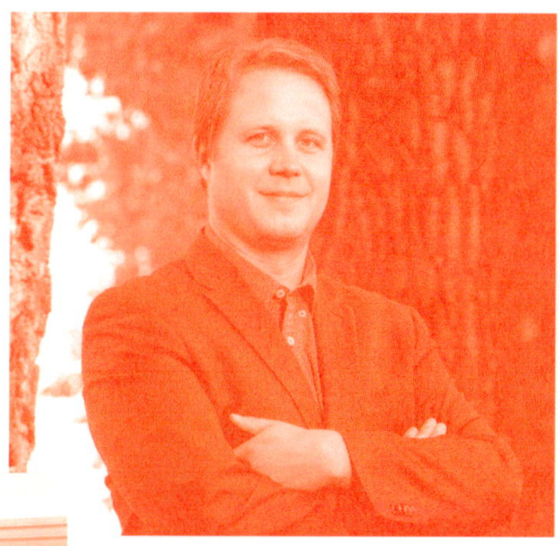
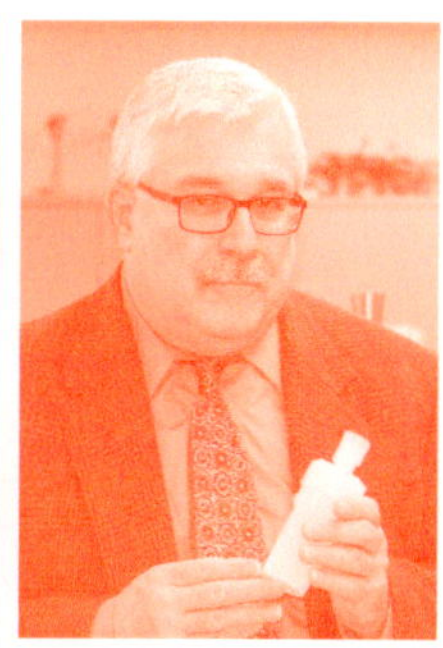
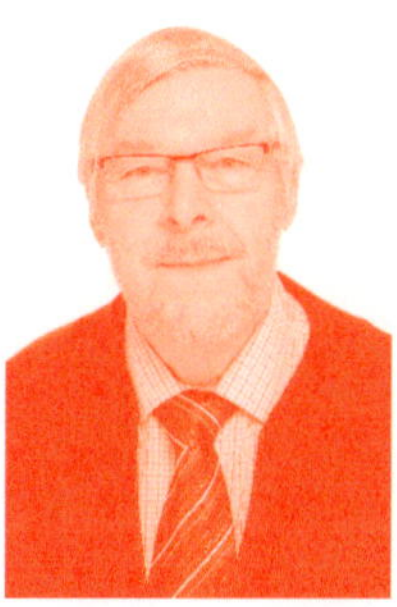
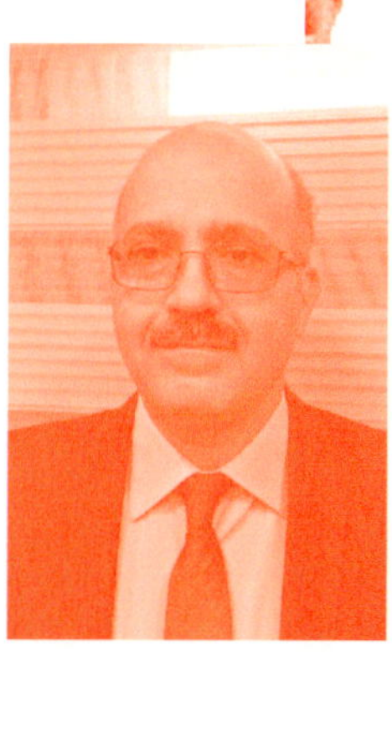
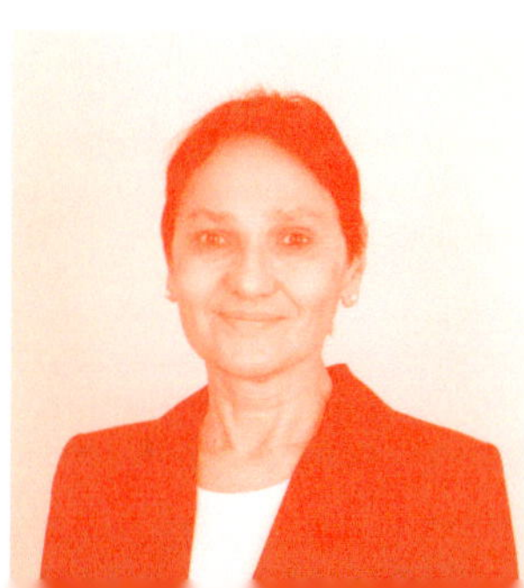
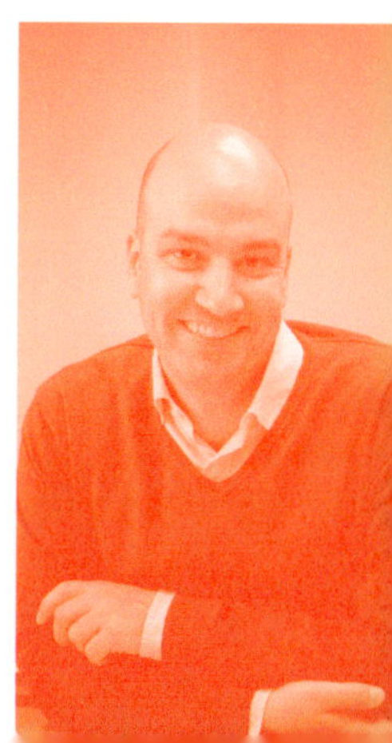

Viruses and Viral Infections in Developing Countries
http://dx.doi.org/10.5772/intechopen.73768
Edited by Snežana Jovanović-Ćupić, Muhammad Abubakar, Ayşe Emel Önal, Muhammad Kashif Saleemi, Ana Božović and Milena Krajnovic

Contributors
Khrisdiana Putri, Widya Asmara, Sitarina Widyarini, Sugiyono Sugiyono, Olatunde Babatunde Akanbi, Anyebe Bernard Onoja, Oluwaseyi Ajagbe, Daniel Benharroch, Yuji Takemoto, Vivek Verma, Dilip C. Nath, María Leticia Saucedo-Mendiola, Elva Marcela Coria-Quiñones, Alejandra Vázquez-Vázquez, Adolfo Padilla Mendiola, María Estela Frías-Zepeda, Jose Luis Ríos- Bañuelos, Jesús Alonso Gándara-Mireles, Tatsuaki Tsuruyama, Norishige Yamada, Shuichiro Ogawa, Jean-Luc Darlix, Muhammad Abubakar, Hugues de Rocquigny, Victor Olusegun Taiwo, Emmanuel Tumininu Obishakin, Pius Stephen Ekong, Israel Joshua Barde, Clement Adebajo Meseko

First published in London, United Kingdom, 2020 by IntechOpen
IntechOpen is the global imprint of INTECHOPEN LIMITED, registered in England and Wales, registration number: 11086078, 7th floor, 10 Lower Thames Street, London, EC3R 6AF, United Kingdom
Printed in Croatia

British Library Cataloguing-in-Publication Data
A catalogue record for this book is available from the British Library

Additional hard and PDF copies can be obtained from orders@intechopen.com

Viruses and Viral Infections in Developing Countries
Edited by Snežana Jovanović-Ćupić, Muhammad Abubakar, Ayşe Emel Önal, Muhammad Kashif Saleemi, Ana Božović and Milena Krajnovic
p. cm.
Print ISBN 978-1-78985-633-0
Online ISBN 978-1-78985-634-7
eBook (PDF) ISBN 978-1-83880-969-0

For EU product safety concerns:
IN TECH d.o.o., Prolaz Marije Krucifikse Kozulić 3, 51000 Rijeka, Croatia, info@intechopen.com or visit our website at intechopen.com.

Meet the editors

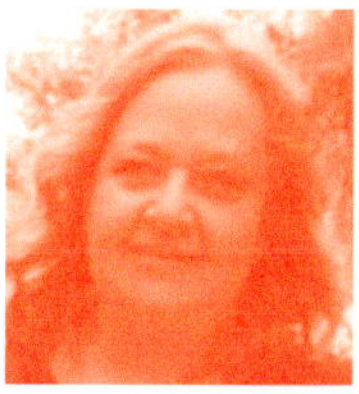

Snežana Jovanović-Ćupić is a research assistant professor in the Institute for Nuclear Sciences-Vinča, University of Belgrade, Belgrade. Snežana received her PhD in Biological Sciences at the Faculty of Biology, University of Belgrade, in 2012. Her research area includes: molecular biology of hepatitis C virus (HCV); genetic variability in HCV and its role in antiviral treatment response; host resistance to HCV infection and influence of immune response to therapy outcome; and association of HCV with hepatocellular carcinoma (including epigenetic background—DNA methylation and microRNA expression). Snežana has published many research articles in peer-reviewed international journals.

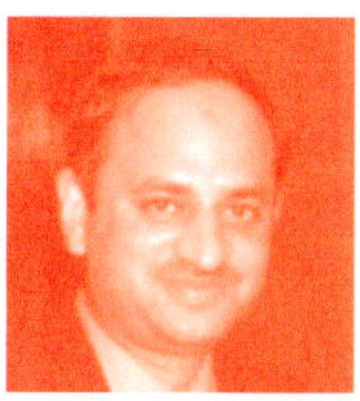

Dr. Muhammad Abubakar, senior scientist from the National Veterinary Laboratory, Islamabad, Pakistan, has over 15 years' experience in various areas of veterinary sciences. His expertise in transboundary animal diseases (TADs) at national and international levels is well known. He has established various diagnostic laboratories for the diagnosis of TADs. He has been involved in the organization and conduct of various trainings for field and laboratory staff. He has published numerous research papers, review articles, and book chapters on different areas of veterinary sciences. He has also worked in academia teaching and research supervising at graduate and undergraduate levels. He is currently supervising two journals in the area of veterinary sciences *(Research Journal for Veterinary Practitioners and Veterinary Sciences and Research and Reviews)* as an editor-in-chief.

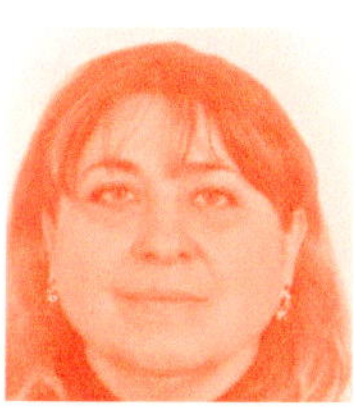

Professor Ayşe Emel Önal, MD, was born in Istanbul in 1960. She graduated from Istanbul University, Istanbul Medical Faculty, in 1985. In 1995, she took a public health specialist diploma with her thesis titled "The relationship between the health problems of elderly teachers living in Istanbul with Daily Life Activities and Instrumental Daily Life Activities" in Istanbul Medical Faculty Department of Public Health. In 2005, she received the title of Public Health Associate Professor at Hacettepe Medical Faculty. Since 1991, she has been working at Istanbul University, Istanbul Medical Faculty Department of Public Health. In 2007, she started work as an associate professor in the Department of Environmental Health. She became a professor in 2011 and continued her duties in Istanbul Medical Faculty Department of Public Health. Since 2013, she has been working as the Head of Environmental Health Science, Department of Public Health, in Istanbul Medical Faculty. In 2014, she began working as the Director of Community Medicine Application and Research Center of Istanbul University. Since 2016, she has been working as the Head of Istanbul University Faculty of

Medicine, Department of Public Health. She is an international book editor and chapter author in three international books and two national books. She has more than 35 international publications in Web of Science; 15 of these are publications in which she is the first name. She has publications in over 100 national journals and papers in international and national congresses. Her H Index is 11. She speaks French and English. Her main research areas are epidemiology, gerontology, and environmental health.

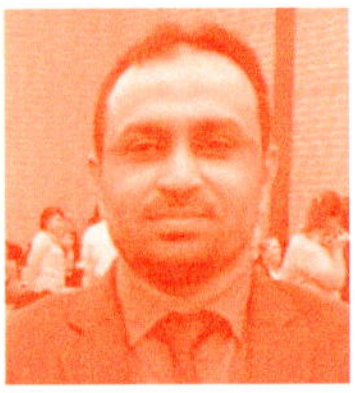

Dr. Muhammad Kashif Saleemi did his DVM in 2001, MSc (Hons) in Veterinary Pathology in 2003 (Silver Medal), and PhD in Veterinary Pathology in 2010 from the Faculty of Veterinary Science, University of Agriculture Faisalabad (UAF), Pakistan. He won a One-Health Fellowship from the US National Academy of Sciences in 2016–17. Currently, he is working as an associate professor (tenured) in the Department of Pathology, UAF. He is a senior academic advisor for the Dean Faculty of Veterinary Science. He is a renowned poultry pathologist in Pakistan. He won the research productivity award for last two years from the Pakistan Council for Science and Technology. He has published 110 research papers in well-reputed international journals having a cumulative impact factor of 165. Currently, he is Associate Editor of the Pakistan Veterinary Journal and a convener of the Poultry Professional Club. He is the National Branch Secretary of WVPA Pakistan. He is also a member of the National Disease Control Committee on Poultry Diseases for the Pakistan Poultry Association.

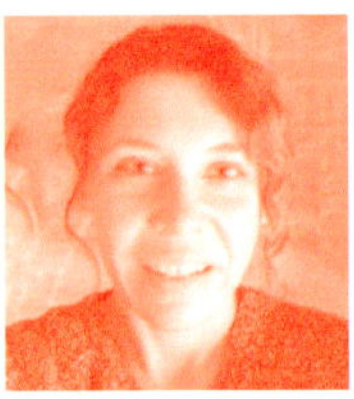

Ana Božović is an assistant research professor at the Vinča Institute of Nuclear Sciences, Serbia. Ana obtained her PhD in 2013 from the University of Belgrade, Serbia. She works at the Molecular Genetics Laboratory at the Vinča Institute of Nuclear Sciences, Serbia. Her research interests include genetic and epigenetic mechanisms of oncogenesis.

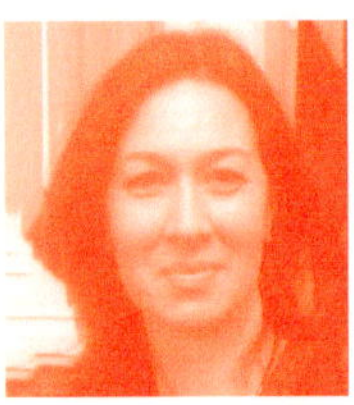

Milena Krajnović is a research assistant professor in the Institute for Nuclear Sciences, Vinča, University of Belgrade, Belgrade. Milena received her PhD in Biological Sciences at the Faculty of Biology, University of Belgrade, in 2013. Her research area includes: molecular oncogenetics, genetic, and epigenetic alterations in human cancers; viruses and cancerogenesis; examination of hepatitis C virus-induced DNA methylation; gene silencing in the host genome and its association with the development of hepatocellular carcinoma and response to antiviral therapy to define potential diagnostic, prognostic, and predictive biomarkers. Milena has published many research articles in peer-reviewed international journals.

Contents

Preface

Viruses are the most prevalent forms of life on Earth. However, our knowledge of viruses is negligible compared to their abundance and impact on human populations and evolution.

This book is divided into three sections. The first section is on specific viral proteins. These proteins have a role in viral replication, protection, and entrance in the host cell. Having in mind the vital roles in the survival of viruses, these proteins are excellent candidates for antiviral therapy. This section also contains information on tumor viruses, as well as human papillomavirus, hepatitis B virus, T-cell leukemia virus, genetic testing, and mutagenesis of murine leukemia retrovirus.

In the second section of the book, the authors focus on avian influenza. Its vast impact on the poultry industry in various developing countries, high infection and mutation rates, and zoonotic potential are the reasons why endangered regions of the world need measures to control these infections.

Finally, the third section of the book is on morbillivirus and its threat to developing countries, where the vaccination coverage is low. Since this virus affects mostly children, there is an urgent need for mass vaccinations. Different regions of the world approach this problem differently. The authors also argue about the oncogenic potential of morbillivirus.

Snežana Jovanović-Ćupić (Editor)
Institute for Nuclear Sciences-Vinca,
Belgrade, Serbia

Muhammad Abubakar (Co-editor(s))
National Veterinary Laboratory,
Islamabad, Pakistan

Ayse Emel Onal
Istanbul Faculty of Medicine,
Istanbul University,
Istanbul, Turkey

Ana Božović and Milena Krajnovic
Institute for Nuclear Sciences-Vinca,
Belgrade, Serbia

Muhammad Kashif Saleemi
University of Agriculture Faisalabad,
Faisalabad, Pakistan

Section 1

Retroviruses, Tumor Viruses and Viral Proteins

Chapter 1

Multiple Functions and Disordered Nature of Nucleocapsid Proteins of Retroviruses and Hepadnaviruses

Jean Luc Darlix and Hugues de Rocquigny

Abstract

This chapter aims at presenting small viral proteins that orchestrate replication of the human immunodeficiency virus type-1 (HIV-1) and the human hepatitis virus (HBV), two canonical examples of small human pathogens. HIV-1 nucleocapsid protein (NC) and the C-terminal domain (CTD) of the HBV core protein (HBc) are essential structural components of the virus capsid ensuring protection of the viral genome; they also chaperone replication of the HIV-1 genomic RNA and the HBV DNA by a reverse-transcription mode, and later, these proteins kick-start virus morphogenesis. HIV-1 NC and HBV CTD belong to the family of intrinsically disordered proteins (IDP), a characteristic rendering possible a large number of molecular interactions. Although these viral proteins share little sequence homologies, they have in common to be rich in basic amino acids and endowed with RNA-binding and chaperoning activities. Similar viral RNA-binding proteins (vRBP) are also encoded for by other virus families, notably flaviviruses, hantaviruses, and coronaviruses. We discuss how these vRBPs function based on the abundant RBP family that plays key physiological roles via multiple interactions with non-coding RNA regulating immune defenses and cell stress. Moreover, these RBPs are flexible molecules allowing dynamic interactions with many RNA and protein partners in a semi-solid milieu favoring biochemical reactions.

Keywords: RBP, HIV, HBV, IDP, RNA chaperoning, molecular crowding

1. Forewords on viruses and RNA chaperones

Viruses that replicate their genome by the process of reverse transcription (RTion) are common in animals, plants, algae, and fungi [1]. These so-called reverse-transcribing viruses have been classified into five different families, namely, *Caulimoviridae*, *Hepadnaviridae*, *Metaviridae*, *Pseudoviridae*, and *Retroviridae* to which was the recently added *Belpaoviridae* [2]. Among these widespread viruses, two are major human pathogens, the human immunodeficiency virus type 1 (HIV-1) and the human hepatitis B virus (HBV).

Retroviruses exist as infectious exogenous RNA viruses as well as endogenous retroelements (ERV) present at high copy numbers in the genome of vertebrates.

Hepadnaviruses can also integrate their genome in the host genome but at a much lower rate [3].

Replication of the genome of these two classes of virus necessitates a reverse transcription step. For HIV-1 the genomic RNA of 9600 nt in length has a structure similar to cellular mRNAs with a 5′ cap and 3′ poly A and contains 9 genes leading to the expression of 15 proteins. Retroviruses replicate their genome by a copy and paste mechanism, whereby the single-stranded positive-sense retroviral genomic RNA is converted into a double-stranded DNA by the virion reverse transcriptase (RT enzyme) [4], subsequently integrated into the host genome [5]. The integrated viral DNA called provirus is expressed by the host transcription machinery to synthesize the full-length viral RNA (FL RNA), which after nuclear export in the cell cytoplasm is translated by the ribosomes to synthesize the major structural proteins and enzymes, the Gag and Gag-Pol precursors. Specific interactions of the genomic RNA with the Gag polyprotein precursor drive Gag polymerization and viral core assembly at the plasma membrane (PM) [6].

For hepadnaviruses the small double-stranded DNA genome in a relaxed circular form (rcDNA) is targeted to the nucleus after virus infection where it is converted into a covalently closed circular form (cccDNA) and expressed by the transcription machinery of the infected cell to synthesize the full-length RNA called pre-genomic RNA (pgRNA) [7]. Upon translation of the pgRNA, the newly made core protein and RT enzyme interact with the pgRNA to synthesize the ds DNA genome. The genome of this virus has unique features such as an extensive overlapping of the genes, namely, 3200 nt with four coding sequences leading to the expression of seven proteins for HBV, and a pseudo-circular structure [8]. In addition several of the HIV and HBV proteins were found to be multifunctional, notably NC, TAT, and VIF protein for HIV and the HBV core protein (HBc) [9, 10].

These two classes of viruses probably emerged during the early Paleozoic Era, some 450–520 million years ago, with a marine origin [11]. The HBVs seem to originate from non-enveloped progenitors called nackednaviruses present in fishes, some 400 million years ago [12].

In addition to an RNA/DNA-dependent DNA polymerase called reverse transcriptase with an associated RNase H activity, these two classes of small viruses encode for a core protein endowed with RNA-binding, unwinding, annealing, and matchmaker activities and the ability to cause the formation of nucleoprotein complexes with a gel-like milieu favoring molecular crowding and biochemical reactions such as reverse transcription.

This chapter will briefly review the multiple roles of the core proteins drawing a parallel between the HIV-1 Gag and the HBV core. In fact these viral core proteins turn out to be much more than a structural component forming a cage enveloping the genome since they provide assistance to the RT-RNase H enzyme at all steps of viral DNA synthesis and then ensure stability of the newly made viral DNA.

Despite common functions in HIV and HBV morphogenesis and replication, the core protein appears much different from Gag on an amino acid sequence basis, but taking a closer look at their activities and functions reveals that these viral proteins are similar.

2. The RNA folding problem and RNA chaperones

The need for RNA chaperones comes from the RNA folding problem whereby RNA molecules have to find their native functional structure in an extremely wide landscape of structures [13]. In fact, RNA chaperones are as diverse and abundant

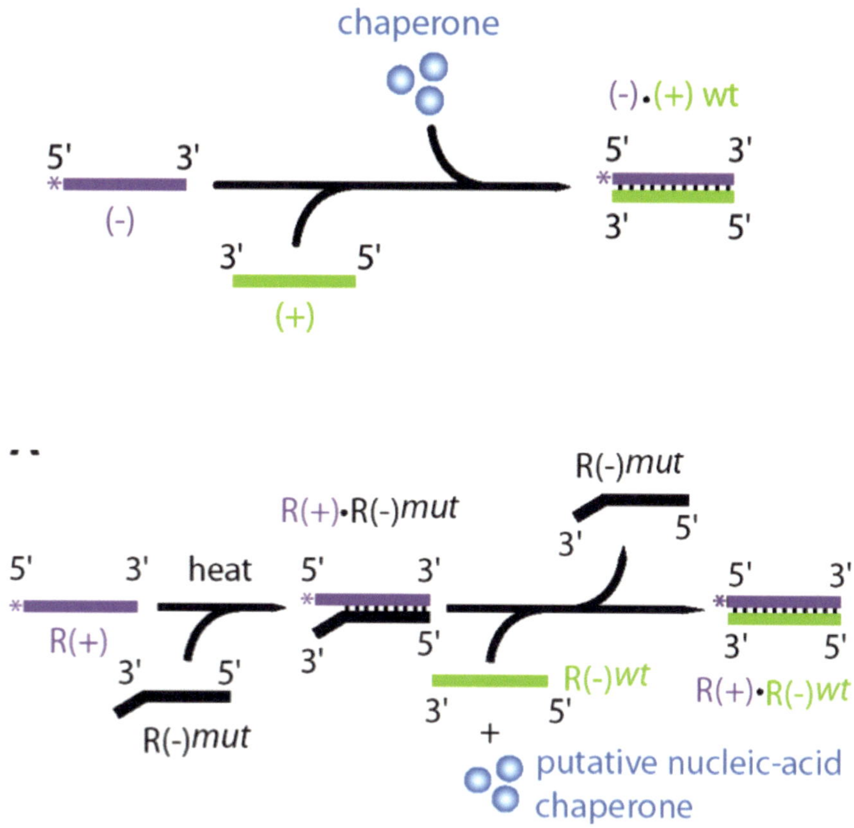

Figure 1.
Standard assays for monitoring the nucleic acid chaperone activity. These in vitro chaperoning assays summarize several properties of nucleic acid chaperone proteins, notably their ability to rapidly anneal complementary nucleic acid sequences (top panel) and favor formation of the most stable duplex, in physiological-like conditions. Bottom panel: R+ and R− sequences represent the 5′ end repeats of the HIV-1 genome of 96 nt in length. R− (mut) contains three mutated residues at its 3′ end in order to generate 3 nt mismatch upon annealing to R+; this was achieved by incubating R+ and R− mut at 66°C for 1 h. Next R− WT is added together with NC protein for 5 min at 30°C. The duplex and ss R− mut were resolved by native gel electrophoresis. Adapted from Darlix et al. [15].

as RNA molecules, coding and noncoding from prokaryotes to eukaryotes [14]. Recent findings highlight the fact that RNA chaperones are disordered in nature and function in a disordered state and do not require ATP as a source of energy to direct RNA folding [13]. Instead RNA chaperones seem to exploit a mechanism of an energy transfer during a rapid on-off RNA-binding kinetics. A number of standard assays are used to monitor RNA chaperoning activity; notably binding, fraying, and annealing of complementary sequences; activation of hammerhead ribozyme-directed cleavage of an RNA substrate; and formation of a dense nucleoprotein complexes. **Figure 1** illustrates assays aimed at describing the influence of NC on DNA strand transfers that occur during the process of reverse transcription resulting in the synthesis of cDNA.

3. The retroviral GAG polyprotein and its multiple roles

The major structural proteins of retroviruses are encoded for by Gag that is formed of several modular domains, namely, Map17, Cap24, NCp7, and p6;

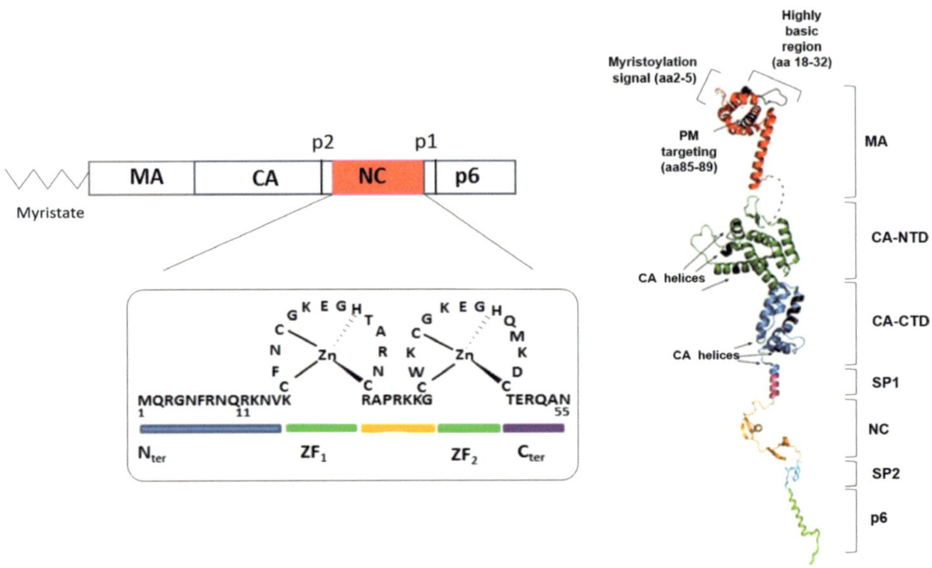

Figure 2.
Structural model of the HIV-1 Gag polyprotein precursor. Left, the different domains of HIV-1 Gag, matrix (Map17), capsid (Cap24), nucleocapsid (NCp7), and p6; two small peptides flanking the NC domain, P2/SP1 and P1/SP2. Right: 2D presentation of the complete Gag Pr55. Adapted from Sundquist and Krausslich [16].

in addition there are two small peptides p1 and p2 flanking NC in the Pr55 gag (**Figure 2**) [16]. The N-terminus is myristoylated, which, together with a row of basic residues within MA, targets Gag to the plasma membrane where assembly takes place [17].

In infected cells the full-length viral RNA is translated by the ribosome machinery to produce the Gag and Gag-Pol polyprotein precursors. The present model of assembly stipulates that newly made Gag molecules accumulate in the cytoplasm, probably in the vicinity of the translating polysomes [18] where they kick-start virus assembly (**Figure 3**); this is achieved through two types of interactions (i) Gag-NC with the 5′ untranslated region (5′ UTR) of FL RNA [19] and (ii) the myristoylated matrix domain with phospholipids of the T-cell membrane [20]. These interactions target the Gag-RNA nucleoprotein complexes to the plasma membrane, causing Gag-oligomer formation; the nucleocapsid domain binds and selects the genomic RNA causing its dimerization and at the same time, together with the capsid domain, boosts Gag multimerization (**Figure 3**). These interactions between Gag and phospholipids as well as RNA lead to virus assembly that takes place at the plasma membrane. Subsequently, virus maturation occurs during the budding process, together with the recruitment of the envelope glycoproteins by the matrix domain [21] (**Figure 3**).

Maturation is a complex process whereby the core of HIV-1 becomes conical and at the same time the genomic RNA dimer is condensed, thus leading to the formation of infectious particles [23]. However most HIV-1 virions and more generally retroviral particles are noninfectious. As a matter of fact, the ratio of infectious virus to noninfectious particles is from 1:10 to 1:10^4 [24, 25]. Thus a majority of particles are noninfectious most probably caused by the loss of envelope proteins, degradation of the genomic RNA, or else correspond to defective-interfering particles (DIP) that can lead to an underestimation of virus infectivity [26].

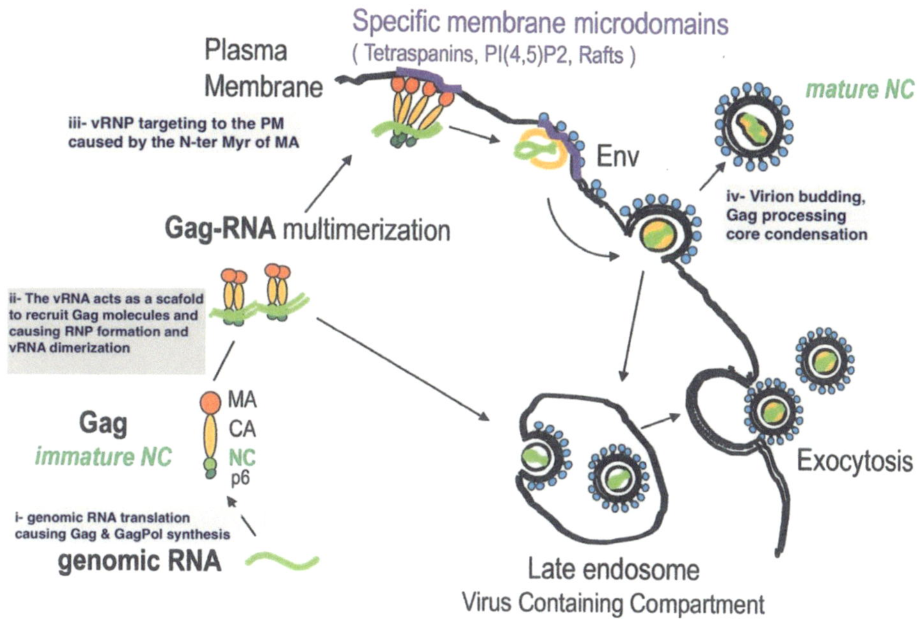

Figure 3.
Schematic representation of virus morphogenesis and the roles of Gag-NC. The genomic RNA is exported from the nucleus and translated by the cell ribosome machinery giving rise to the production of the Gag and Gag-Pol precursors. Gag-NC binds the packaging signal at the 5′ end of the genomic RNA causing the formation of the viral nucleoprotein complex (vRNP) and dimerization of the genomic RNA. Such vRNP are targeted to the plasma membrane where they accumulate to form immature viral particles. Next, the Gag molecules are processed by the viral protease causing core condensation. Adapted from Muriaux and Darlix [22].

4. Characteristics of retroviral nucleocapsid proteins

Retroviral nucleocapsid proteins are small basic proteins with either one (MuLV, gammaretrovirus) or two CCHC zinc fingers (HIV and FIV, lentiviruses; RSV an *Alpharetrovirus*) (**Table 1**). The zinc fingers are structured upon Zn^{2+} binding (in red), while the flanking domains are disordered and basic. Therefore, these viral proteins are members of the large family of intrinsically disordered proteins/intrinsically disordered protein domains (IDPDs) [27–29]. Of note all these NC proteins are endowed with RNA-binding and chaperoning activities as shown using in vitro reconstituted systems [15, 30–32]. Other important characteristics are the ability of these NC proteins to cause the formation of nucleoprotein complexes capable of recruiting enzymes such as reverse transcriptase and integrase (IN) [33]. In this gel-like milieu, molecular crowding can take place, thus facilitating enzymatic reactions, such as cDNA synthesis by RT and integration by IN. Along this line, NC protein interacts with RT improving the fidelity of cDNA synthesis by several different ways: (i) inhibition of self-primed initiation of cDNA synthesis, (ii) chaperoning the obligatory minus- and plus-stranded transfers for the synthesis of the LTR flanking the viral DNA (**Figure 1**), and (iii) improving the processivity of RT as well as its excision repair activity resulting in a much higher fidelity of viral DNA synthesis (**Figure 1** on chaperoning assays).

How is this achieved? According to Uversky, protein-RNA interfaces are most probably very large with the concomitant implications of basic, hydrophobic, and aromatic residues engaged, respectively, in ionic, hydrophobic, and intercalating interactions [34–36]. The interactions between NC and RT are poorly understood, but they appear to necessitate the RNA template as the scaffolding agent [37, 38].

HIV-1 NCp7:	MQRGNFRNQRKMVK CFNCGKEGHTARNC RAPRKKG CWKCGKEGHQMKDC TERQANFL
HIV-1 NCp7-SP2:	MQRGNFRNQRKNVK CFNCGKEGHTARNC RAPRKKG CWKCGKEGHQMKDC TERQANFLGKIWPSYKGRPGN
FIV NCp8:	ALTKVQTVQAKGPGPV CFNCKRPGHLARQC REVKK CNKCGKPGHLAANC WQGGKKNQGNW
RSV NCp12:	AVVNRERDGQTGSGGRARGL CYTCGSPGHYQAQC PKKRKSGNSRER CQLCDGMGHNAKQC RRRDGNQGQRPGKGLSSGSWPVSEQPAV
MuLV NCp10:	ATVVSGQKQDRQDRQGERRRSQLDRDQ CAYCKEKGHWAKDC PKKPRGPRGPRPQELL
Ty3 NCp9:	TVRTRRSYNKPMSNHRNRRNNNASREECIKRNRL CFYCKKEGHRLNEC RARKASSNRS
HBV core (CTD):	TTV VRRR G RSPRRR TPSP RRRRS QSP RRRRS QSRESQC

Table 1.
Sequences of retroviral nucleocapsid proteins and the C-terminus of HBV core protein. The one-letter code has been used, and the basic domains are in black, while the CX2CX4HX2C zinc fingers are in red. Note the low complexity basic domains flanking the NC zinc fingers. For the yeast retrotransposon Ty3, note the zinc finger essential for TY3 retrotransposition and the low complexity flanking sequences. The C-terminal domain of the HBV core protein has four R-rich sequences and is of low complexity.

In that respect the RTp66 subunit with its active site appears to be extremely flexible with notably a large template-binding pocket. These observations favor the notion that the viral proteins NC and RT and the template RNA making up the replication machine exhibit a flexible nature in an active nucleoprotein complex in agreement with the proposal of Uversky [29]. These in vitro and ex vivo studies on retroviral Gag polyproteins and NC proteins have essentially been carried out using HIV-1 (**Table 1**); additional experiments performed with *Alpharetrovirus* RSV NCp12 with two zinc fingers flanked by basic residues; NCp10 of the gammaretrovirus MuLV, with a unique zinc finger flanked by basic residues; and of the yeast retrotransposon Ty3 NCp9, with a unique zinc finger and basic residues, gave very similar results with respect to RNA binding, chaperoning, and ribonucleoprotein complex formation in vitro (**Table 1**).

5. The core protein of HBV and its roles in virus assembly and viral DNA synthesis

HBV is an enveloped virus with a 3.2 kb partially double-stranded DNA genome referred to as rcDNA [7] that is synthesized by reverse transcription of the pgRNA [39]. The core protein contains 183–185 residues corresponding to two domains (**Figure 4**): the N-terminus (NTD) (residues 1–140) that oligomerizes in a capsid structure linked by a flexible sequence to the basic C-terminal domain (CTD) (residues 150–183) [40, 42, 43]. The core CTD interacts with nucleic acids and is endowed with nucleic acids annealing, matchmaker, and aggregating activities [8, 44].

The HBV core protein orchestrates virus assembly to form an icosahedral capsid [54] (**Figure 5**). During assembly, HBc specifically recognizes the Pol-pgRNA complex [55], promotes its packaging into nascent particles, and assists rcDNA synthesis by the viral RT and cccDNA maintenance [56–58] (for review see Seeger and Mason [59]). The processes of RTion and capsid maturation are regulated by CTD phosphorylation/dephosphorylation [41, 60–62] together with structural rearrangements of the capsid structure [63–65]; this influences capsid trafficking in virus-producing cells and is driven by an unknown mechanism the viral ribonucleoprotein (vRNP) complex to the nucleus and thus the formation of cccDNA. Else the vRNP is targeted to cellular compartments where they interact with the envelope proteins

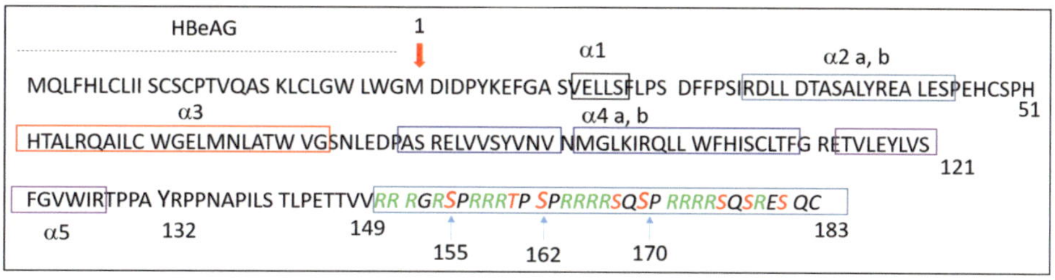

Figure 4.
HBV core primary sequence. The core protein is divided into two parts: the N-terminus (1–140) and the C-terminus (150–183). The N-terminus is sufficient in vitro for the process of self-assembly [8]. NTD monomer contains a series of five α helices, the third and the fourth helices associate in a four-helix bundle giving the characteristic spikes at the surface of assembled capsids [40]. The C-terminus contains arginine residues essential for the interaction of core with NA an activity that is regulated by the phosphorylation of the seven serine residues [41]. The effect of mutations in the flexible linker between NTD and CTD (141–149) suggests that the orientation of NTD respective to CTD is essential in the multistage process of HBV replication [42].

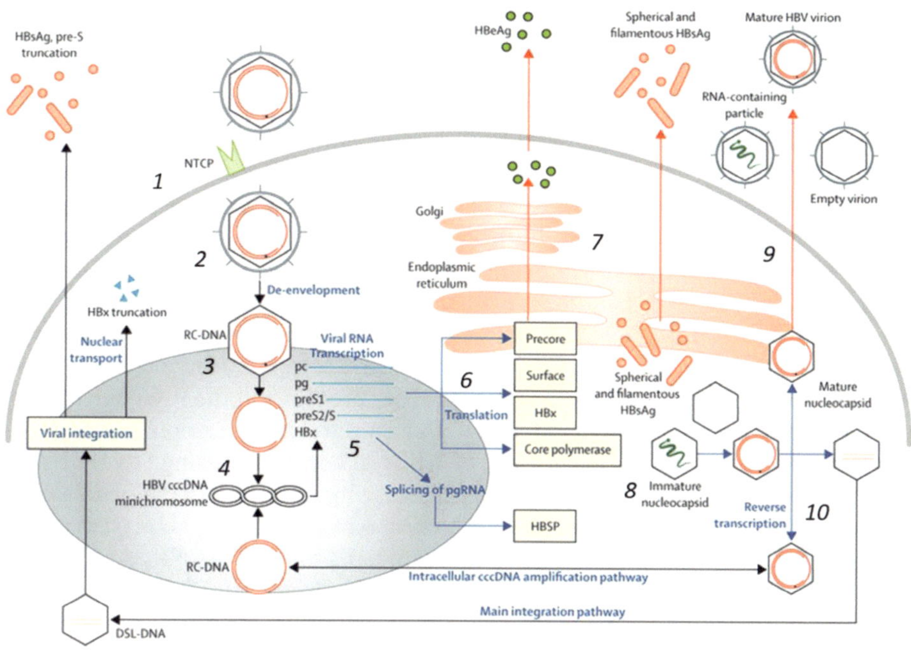

Figure 5.
HBV replication cycle. (1) Virus attachment to the sodium-taurocholate cotransporting polypeptide (NTCP) and entry [45]. (2) Nucleocapsid release in the cytoplasm upon fusion of the cellular and viral membranes and trafficking to the nucleus [43]. This traffic is probably mediated by the CTD containing NLSs [46]. (3) Nuclear pore attachment of the nucleocapsid and release of the rcDNA (relaxed circular) into the nucleus with reorganization of the capsid [47]. (4) Conversion of the rcDNA into cccDNA (covalently closed circular DNA) and formation of a nucleosome-bound minichromosome, possibly associated with HBx, core protein, histone, and nonhistone cellular proteins [7]. (5) Transcription generating the pre-genomic RNA, precore RNA, preS1/preS2/S mRNAs, and HBx mRNA [48]. (6) Synthesis of the viral proteins by the cell machinery. (7) Production of HBeAg and assembly of S alone with some L protein giving rise to subviral particles. (8) Formation of empty capsids or pgRNA-Pol containing capsids with immature nucleocapsids. Reverse transcription of pgRNA to generate rcDNA is concomitant with the maturation of the nucleocapsid. (9) Both empty and mature particles are embedded by L and S proteins and produced in the supernatant [49]. The egress of particles necessitates the endosomal sorting complexes required for transport (ESCRT) [50] even though naked capsids were shown to be released through the ALIX pathway [51]. (10) Alternatively, the rcDNA-containing particles recycle to the nucleus, amplifying the cccDNA copy numbers [52]. Adapted from Revill et al. [53].

promoting virus egress [43, 66, 67] (for review see Blondot et al. [68]). HBV secretion remains a challenging issue since different types of viral particles are found in the circulating blood of patients. Despite a heterogeneous distribution from patients to patients, it is estimated that most of the particles are consisting of the sole envelope proteins (HBsAg) as sphere and filaments also referred to as Australian antigen (10^{14}/ml), empty particles (without genome, 10^{11}/ml), RNA-containing virions (10^{6}/ml), and complete infectious particles (Dane particles, 10^{9}/ml) [49]. The low amount Dane particles remain unclear, and it has been proposed that reverse transcription of the pgRNA triggers a structural change of the capsid (maturation signal), which in turn causes the envelopment and secretion of complete infectious virions [65, 69]. More recently the group of Hu et al. proposed a two-signal model, the first one exposed in the empty particles at the level of the NTD-CTD linker resulting in an interaction with the S protein and the second one exposed in maturate particles at the level of the MBD (matrix-binding domain) to cause an interaction with the L envelope [70, 71] (for review see Liu and Hu [72]). Even though the molecular bases of these two domains remain to be clarified, they both lie on the capsid structure in agreement with the large effect of capsid envelopment by single-point mutations around the hydrophobic pocket in the center of the spikes [73–76]. Thus the envelopment of the vRNP is closely linked to the HBc protein that represents a critical factor in virus replication and as a matter of fact, a target in the search for antiviral molecules [77, 78].

6. The CTD of HBV core protein has nucleic acid chaperone activity

The nucleic acid chaperone activity of the CTD was first suggested by the group of Loeb [66] and of Zlotnick [79]. In the first case, they followed the strand transfer of the initial (−) DNA from the 5′ ε bulge to the 3′ DR1 sequence and (−) DNA elongation. This suggests that the core protein has a nucleic chaperone activity similar to retroviral NC [30, 32, 34, 80, 81]. In the second case, using core constructs mimicking the unphosphorylated or phosphorylated core, they found a correlation between the number of positive charge in the core protein and the RNA density suggesting that the core protein induced RNA structural modification.

The RNA/DNA chaperoning activity of HBc was confirmed using DNA-DNA hybridization and hammerhead ribozyme cleavage in vitro [56]. In the first assay, authors followed the annealing of the DNA version of HIV TAR. This sequence is located in the 5′ end of HIV genome. In addition to its role in the RNA transcription with TAT protein [82, 83], this sequence is essential for the (−) single-stranded transfer along the RT-dependent synthesis of HIV DNA [30, 32, 34, 81]. Interestingly they compared assembled and disassembled HBc particles and found that dissembled HBc was more efficient in DNA duplex formation. Using a series of peptides, they found that this chaperoning activity maps at the CTD and required the four stretches of basic residues (**Table 1**). When a peptide is containing phosphorylated serine residues at the positions 155, 162, and 170, considered as the three major serine phosphorylation sites, the DNA annealing activity was progressively reduced as a function of the number of phosphorylation sites. Similar results were obtained with the hammerhead ribozyme cleavage assays [27] (**Figure 6**).

The role of HBc nucleic acid annealing and matchmaker activities was assessed using viral particles. Therefore, a plasmid expressing HBV genome with a stop codon in the HBc ORF was cotransfected with a plasmid expressing core in agreement with the fact that HBV competent for the replication can be obtained by trans-complementation assays [84, 85]. Mutations shown to decrease HBc in vitro activity gave rise to an important decrease of HBV DNA synthesis and a loss of viral replication. These results support the notion that HBc has nucleic acid chaperone activity essential for minus-stranded and plus-stranded DNA synthesis along the replication cycle. Nevertheless, the defect observed in viral DNA synthesis could

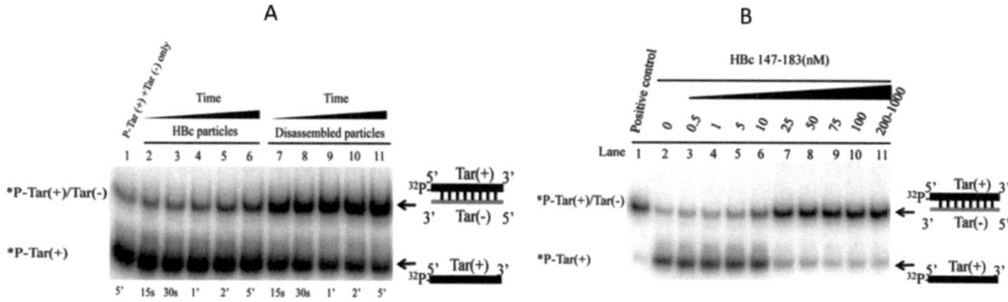

Figure 6.
Annealing activity of HBc and HBc (147–183). (A) TAR(+)/TAR(−) annealing activity of HBc particles (left) and HBc protein (right) as a function of time. TAR(+) was ^{32}P labelled using T4 polynucleotide kinase, purified by PAGE and recovered by ethanol precipitation. TAR(+) and TAR(−) were mixed with HBc in NaCl-containing TRIS buffer. At time points 15 s to 5 min HBc was removed by a proteinase K treatment and reaction stopped by addition of EDTA. TAR DNAs were resolved by 8% PAGE and gels were dried and autoradiographed. (B) TAR(+)/TAR(−) annealing activity of the HBc CTD peptide. This assay was performed as described above at various concentrations for 5 min. Panels A and B were extracted from ***Figures 1*** *and* ***3*** *of [56].*

originate from a defect of HBc assembly [86, 87], RNA encapsidation [88, 89], HBc trafficking [46, 68, 90], or HBc maturation/single-stranded blocking model [65, 69–71] since all these steps require the arginine residues of the C-terminus.

7. Concluding remarks and questions

As for retroviruses that are widespread in living organisms and can rapidly and efficiently circulate and spread in animals, even crossing species barriers, the small basic protein called NC has multiple functions in virus structure, replication, and dissemination. Indeed, NC protein is a helper factor for the RT enzyme and its associated RNAse H activity and also for the integrase enzyme. NC is indeed a chaperoning factor required from the start to the end of viral DNA synthesis as well as for the recruitment of cofactors required for transport (**Figure 7**). Also they are considered as membrane-less organelles that play key roles in cells such as fine tuning of gene expression, translation, and immune controls via noncoding RNAs. Furthermore, NC is a key factor for driving the recombination reactions fuelling the genetic diversity of the newly made viral particles.

The HBV C-terminal domain (C-ter) appears to play multiple roles in virus replication in a manner similar to the retroviral NC protein, by chaperoning genome replication ensuring the fidelity of the viral DNA synthesis and its stability once it is complete.

There are many questions on how do such viral nucleoprotein complexes function.

One concerns the process of reverse transcription, i.e., how does the RT enzyme copy the RNA molecule coated by hundreds of such highly basic protein molecules? Another one deals with the permeability of these viral nucleoprotein ensembles [91], i.e., the accessibility of cofactors that can be helper or restriction factors such as cytidine and adenosine deaminases, apolipoprotein B-editing catalytic subunit (APOBEC) [92], or adenosine deaminase acting on RNA-1 (ADAR1) that was recently shown to inhibit HBV replication by enhancing microRNA-122 processing [93]. Furthermore, the recruitment of restriction factors is not an on-off process since a limited accessibility appears to take place for both HIV and HBV, impacting on the genetic diversity of the virus that is a major issue in antiviral treatments [94, 95].

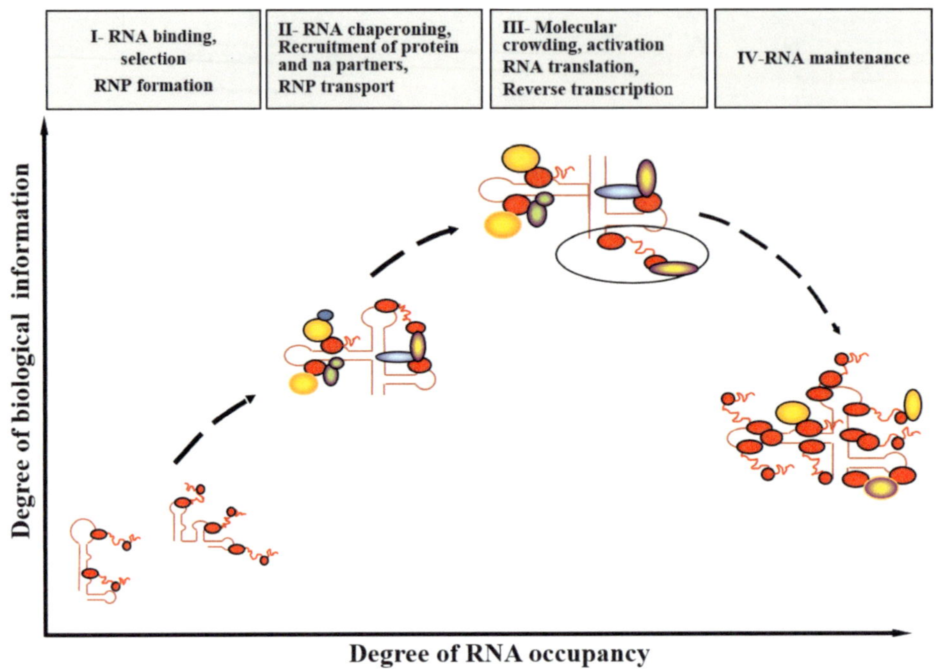

Figure 7.
Formation of nucleoprotein complexes and functions according to the degree of RNA occupancy. With the increasing level of RNA occupancy by the chaperone protein, functions go from selection of the genomic RNA (I), its dimerization (II), to the complete process of reverse transcription (III) or else are targeted to RNP granules (IV).

On a more general basis, vRBP's with chaperoning activities are widespread in the virus world, since they are, for example, encoded for by other virus families such as flaviviruses, notably the core proteins of HCV and dengue viruses, the N protein of coronaviruses and hantaviruses, and the delta antigen of the HDV viroid [96–103]. In addition, unpublished data show that the N protein of influenza virus has also chaperone activity.

Similar RNA chaperone proteins are found in bacteriophages of the *Leviviridae* family where they regulate vRNA translation and assembly [104]. Also a closer look at the replication of the Q-beta genomic RNA by the viral replicase reveals the chaperoning contribution of the host factors EF-Tu and Ts. These data favor the notion that RNA chaperones may also influence protein conformation and enzymatic activity, raising the possibility that such proteins are Janus chaperones [28, 105, 106].

Acknowledgements

Personal (JLD) thanks are due to my spouse Anne Napoly and to Yves Mély (Faculty of Pharmacy, Strasbourg) for their continuous support during the past 12 months and to Lada Bozic for her kind understanding. Supports from INSERM, ANRS, and Philippe Roingeard (Faculty of Medicine, Tours) are acknowledged (HdR).

Author details

Jean Luc Darlix[1,3*†] and Hugues de Rocquigny[2*†]

1 Laboratory of Bioimaging and Pathologies (LBP), UMR 7021, Faculty of Pharmacy, University of Strasbourg, Illkirch, France

2 Morphogenèse et Antigénicité du VIH et des Virus des Hépatites, Inserm—U1259 MAVIVH, Tours Cedex 1, France

3 Centre National de la Recherche Scientifique, Paris, France

*Address all correspondence to: jldarlix@gmail.com
and hderocquigny@univ-tours.fr

† These authors contributed equally to this work.

References

[1] Hayward A, Cornwallis CK, Jern P. Pan-vertebrate comparative genomics unmasks retrovirus macroevolution. Proceedings of the National Academy of Sciences of the United States of America. 2015;**112**:464-469. DOI: 10.1073/pnas.1414980112

[2] Krupovic M, Blomberg J, Coffin JM, Dasgupta I, Hung F, Geering AD, et al. Ortervirales: New virus order unifying five families of reverse-transcribing viruses. Journal of Virology. 2018;**92**:1-5. DOI: 10.1128/JVI.00515-18

[3] Budzinska MA, Shackel NA, Urban S, Tu T. Cellular genomic sites of hepatitis B virus DNA integration. Genes. 2018;**9**:365-383. DOI: 10.3390/genes9070365

[4] Poeschla E. The importance of becoming double-stranded: Innate immunity and the kinetic model of HIV-1 central plus strand synthesis. Virology. 2013;**441**:1-11. DOI: 10.1016/j.virol.2013.03.010

[5] Lesbats P, Engelman AN, Cherepanov P. Retroviral DNA integration. Chemical Reviews. 2016;**116**:12730-12757. DOI: 10.1021/acs.chemrev.6b00125

[6] Ferrer M, Henriet S, Chamontin C, Laine S, Mougel M. From cells to virus particles: Quantitative methods to monitor RNA packaging. Viruses. 2016;**8**:239-255. DOI: 10.3390/v8080239

[7] Nassal M. HBV cccDNA: Viral persistence reservoir and key obstacle for a cure of chronic hepatitis B. Gut. 2015;**64**:1972-1984. DOI: 10.1136/gutjnl-2015-309809

[8] Venkatakrishnan B, Zlotnick A. The structural biology of hepatitis B virus: Form and function. Annual Review of Virology. 2016;**3**:429-451. DOI: 10.1146/annurev-virology-110615-042238

[9] Faust TB, Binning JM, Gross JD, Frankel AD. Making sense of multifunctional proteins: Human immunodeficiency virus type 1 accessory and regulatory proteins and connections to transcription. Annual Review of Virology. 2017;**4**:241-260. DOI: 10.1146/annurev-virology-101416-041654

[10] McNaughton AL, D'Arienzo V, Ansari MA, Lumley SF, Littlejohn M, Revill P, et al. Insights from deep sequencing of the HBV genome-unique, tiny, and misunderstood. Gastroenterology. 2019;**156**:384-399. DOI: 10.1053/j.gastro.2018.07.058

[11] Han GZ, Worobey M. An endogenous foamy-like viral element in the coelacanth genome. PLoS Pathogens. 2012;**8**:e1002790. DOI: 10.1371/journal.ppat.1002790

[12] Lauber C, Seitz S, Mattei S, Suh A, Beck J, Herstein J, et al. Deciphering the origin and evolution of hepatitis B viruses by means of a family of non-enveloped fish viruses. Cell Host & Microbe. 2017;**22**:387-399.e386. DOI: 10.1016/j.chom.2017.07.019

[13] Semrad K, Green R, Schroeder R. RNA chaperone activity of large ribosomal subunit proteins from *Escherichia coli*. RNA. 2004;**10**:1855-1860. DOI: 10.1261/rna.7121704

[14] Rajkowitsch L, Chen D, Stampfl S, Semrad K, Waldsich C, Mayer O, et al. RNA chaperones, RNA annealers and RNA helicases. RNA Biology. 2007;**4**:118-130. DOI: 10.4161/rna.4.3.5445

[15] Darlix JL, Lapadat-Tapolsky M, de Rocquigny H, Roques BP. First glimpses at structure-function relationships of the nucleocapsid protein of retroviruses. Journal of Molecular Biology. 1995;**254**:523-537

[16] Sundquist WI, Krausslich HG. HIV-1 assembly, budding, and maturation. Cold Spring Harbor Perspectives in Medicine. 2012;**2**:a006924. DOI: 10.1101/cshperspect.a006924

[17] Kerviel A, Thomas A, Chaloin L, Favard C, Muriaux D. Virus assembly and plasma membrane domains: Which came first? Virus Research. 2013;**171**:332-340. DOI: 10.1016/j.virusres.2012.08.014

[18] Scarlata S, Carter C. Role of HIV-1 Gag domains in viral assembly. Biochimica et Biophysica Acta (BBA)—Biomembranes. 2003;**1614**:62-72. DOI: 10.1016/S0005-2736(03)00163-9

[19] Mailler E, Bernacchi S, Marquet R, Paillart JC, Vivet-Boudou V, Smyth RP. The life-cycle of the HIV-1 Gag-RNA complex. Viruses. 2016;**8**:248-267. DOI: 10.3390/v8090248

[20] Lingappa JR, Reed JC, Tanaka M, Chutiraka K, Robinson BA. How HIV-1 Gag assembles in cells: Putting together pieces of the puzzle. Virus Research. 2014;**193**:89-107. DOI: 10.1016/j.virusres.2014.07.001

[21] Lee S-K, Potempa M, Swanstrom R. The choreography of HIV-1 proteolytic processing and virion assembly. The Journal of Biological Chemistry. 2012;**287**:40867-40874. DOI: 10.1074/jbc.R112.399444

[22] Muriaux D, Darlix JL. Properties and functions of the nucleocapsid protein in virus assembly. RNA Biology. 2010;**7**:744-753. DOI: 10.4161/rna.7.6.14065

[23] Campbell EM, Hope TJ. HIV-1 capsid: The multifaceted key player in HIV-1 infection. Nature Reviews Microbiology. 2015;**13**:471-483. DOI: 10.1038/nrmicro3503

[24] Dimitrov DS, Willey RL, Sato H, Chang LJ, Blumenthal R, Martin MA. Quantitation of human immunodeficiency virus type 1 infection kinetics. Journal of Virology. 1993;**67**:2182-2190

[25] Rusert P, Fischer M, Joos B, Leemann C, Kuster H, Flepp M, et al. Quantification of infectious HIV-1 plasma viral load using a boosted in vitro infection protocol. Virology. 2004;**326**:113-129. DOI: 10.1016/j.virol.2004.05.022

[26] Klasse PJ. Molecular determinants of the ratio of inert to infectious virus particles. Progress in Molecular Biology and Translational Science. 2015;**129**:285-326. DOI: 10.1016/bs.pmbts.2014.10.012

[27] Herschlag D. RNA chaperones and the RNA folding problem. The Journal of Biological Chemistry. 1995;**270**:20871-20874

[28] Kovacs D, Rakacs M, Agoston B, Lenkey K, Semrad K, Schroeder R, et al. Janus chaperones: Assistance of both RNA- and protein-folding by ribosomal proteins. FEBS Letters. 2009;**583**:88-92. DOI: 10.1016/j.febslet.2008.11.049

[29] Uversky VN. Intrinsic disorder-based protein interactions and their modulators. Current Pharmaceutical Design. 2013;**19**:4191-4213. DOI: 10.2174/1381612811319230005

[30] Godet J, Mely Y. Biophysical studies of the nucleic acid chaperone properties of the HIV-1 nucleocapsid protein. RNA Biology. 2010;**7**:687-699. DOI: 10.4161/rna.7.6.13616

[31] Levin JG, Guo J, Rouzina I, Musier-Forsyth K. Nucleic acid chaperone activity of HIV-1 nucleocapsid protein: Critical role in reverse transcription and molecular mechanism. Progress in Nucleic Acid Research and Molecular Biology. 2005;**80**:217-286

[32] Rein A. Nucleic acid chaperone activity of retroviral Gag proteins. RNA Biology. 2010;**7**:700-705

[33] Summers MF, Karn J. Special issue: Structural and molecular biology of HIV. Journal of Molecular Biology. 2011;**410**:489-490. DOI: 10.1016/j.jmb.2011.05.001

[34] Darlix JL, de Rocquigny H, Mauffret O, Mely Y. Retrospective on the all-in-one retroviral nucleocapsid protein. Virus Research. 2014;**193**:2-15. DOI: 10.1016/j.virusres.2014.05.011

[35] Hentze MW, Castello A, Schwarzl T, Preiss T. A brave new world of RNA-binding proteins. Nature Reviews Molecular Cell Biology. 2018;**19**:327-341. DOI: 10.1038/nrm.2017.130

[36] Rene B, Mauffret O, Fosse P. Retroviral nucleocapsid proteins and DNA strand transfers. Biochimie Open. 2018;7:10-25. DOI: 10.1016/j.biopen.2018.07.001

[37] Druillennec S, Caneparo A, de Rocquigny H, Roques BP. Evidence of interactions between the nucleocapsid protein NCp7 and the reverse transcriptase of HIV-1. The Journal of Biological Chemistry. 1999;**274**:11283-11288

[38] Lener D, Tanchou V, Roques BP, Le Grice SF, Darlix JL. Involvement of HIV-I nucleocapsid protein in the recruitment of reverse transcriptase into nucleoprotein complexes formed in vitro. The Journal of Biological Chemistry. 1998;**273**:33781-33786

[39] Nassal M. Hepatitis B viruses: Reverse transcription a different way. Virus Research. 2008;**134**:235-249. DOI: 10.1016/j.virusres.2007.12.024

[40] Wynne SA, Crowther RA, Leslie AG. The crystal structure of the human hepatitis B virus capsid. Molecular Cell. 1999;**3**:771-780

[41] Heger-Stevic J, Zimmermann P, Lecoq L, Bottcher B, Nassal M. Hepatitis B virus core protein phosphorylation: Identification of the SRPK1 target sites and impact of their occupancy on RNA binding and capsid structure. PLoS Pathogens. 2018;**14**:e1007488. DOI: 10.1371/journal.ppat.1007488

[42] Liu K, Luckenbaugh L, Ning X, Xi J, Hu J. Multiple roles of core protein linker in hepatitis B virus replication. PLoS Pathogens. 2018;**14**:e1007085. DOI: 10.1371/journal.ppat.1007085

[43] Gallucci L, Kann M. Nuclear import of hepatitis B virus capsids and genome. Viruses. 2017;**9**:21-40. DOI: 10.3390/v9010021

[44] Diab A, Foca A, Zoulim F, Durantel D, Andrisani O. The diverse functions of the hepatitis B core/capsid protein (HBc) in the viral life cycle: Implications for the development of HBc-targeting antivirals. Antiviral Research. 2018;**149**:211-220. DOI: 10.1016/j.antiviral.2017.11.015

[45] Yan H, Zhong G, Xu G, He W, Jing Z, Gao Z, et al. Sodium taurocholate cotransporting polypeptide is a functional receptor for human hepatitis B and D virus. eLife. 2012;**1**:e00049. DOI: 10.7554/eLife.00049

[46] Li HC, Huang EY, Su PY, Wu SY, Yang CC, Lin YS, et al. Nuclear export and import of human hepatitis B virus capsid protein and particles. PLoS Pathogens. 2010;**6**:e1001162. DOI: 10.1371/journal.ppat.1001162

[47] Rabe B, Delaleau M, Bischof A, Foss M, Sominskaya I, Pumpens P, et al. Nuclear entry of hepatitis B virus capsids involves disintegration to protein dimers followed by nuclear reassociation to capsids. PLoS Pathogens. 2009;**5**:e1000563. DOI: 10.1371/journal.ppat.1000563

[48] Block TM, Guo H, Guo J-T. Molecular virology of hepatitis B virus for clinicians. Clinics in Liver Disease. 2007;**11**:685-706. DOI: 10.1016/j.cld.2007.08.002

[49] Hu J, Liu K. Complete and incomplete hepatitis B virus particles: Formation, function, and application. Viruses. 2017;**9**:56-73. DOI: 10.3390/v9030056

[50] Watanabe T, Sorensen EM, Naito A, Schott M, Kim S, Ahlquist P. Involvement of host cellular multivesicular body functions in hepatitis B virus budding. Proceedings of the National Academy of Sciences of the United States of America. 2007;**104**:10205-10210. DOI: 10.1073/pnas.0704000104

[51] Bardens A, Doring T, Stieler J, Prange R. Alix regulates egress of hepatitis B virus naked capsid particles in an ESCRT-independent manner. Cellular Microbiology. 2011;**13**:602-619. DOI: 10.1111/j.1462-5822.2010.01557.x

[52] Prange R. Host factors involved in hepatitis B virus maturation, assembly, and egress. Medical Microbiology and Immunology. 2012;**201**:449-461. DOI: 10.1007/s00430-012-0267-9

[53] Revill PA, Chisari FV, Block JM, Dandri M, Gehring AJ, Guo H, et al. A global scientific strategy to cure hepatitis B. The Lancet Gastroenterology and Hepatology. 2019;**4**:545-558. DOI: 10.1016/s2468-1253(19)30119-0

[54] Zlotnick A, Venkatakrishnan B, Tan Z, Lewellyn E, Turner W, Francis S. Core protein: A pleiotropic keystone in the HBV lifecycle. Antiviral Research. 2015;**121**:82-93. DOI: 10.1016/j.antiviral.2015.06.020

[55] Lott L, Beames B, Notvall L, Lanford RE. Interaction between hepatitis B virus core protein and reverse transcriptase. Journal of Virology. 2000;**74**:11479-11489

[56] Chu TH, Liou AT, Su PY, Wu HN, Shih C. Nucleic acid chaperone activity associated with the arginine-rich domain of human hepatitis B virus core protein. Journal of Virology. 2014;**88**:2530-2543. DOI: 10.1128/JVI.03235-13

[57] Hirsch RC, Lavine JE, Chang LJ, Varmus HE, Ganem D. Polymerase gene products of hepatitis B viruses are required for genomic RNA packaging as well as for reverse transcription. Nature. 1990;**344**:552-555. DOI: 10.1038/344552a0

[58] Nassal M, Junker-Niepmann M, Schaller H. Translational inactivation of RNA function: Discrimination against a subset of genomic transcripts during HBV nucleocapsid assembly. Cell. 1990;**63**:1357-1363

[59] Seeger C, Mason WS. Molecular biology of hepatitis B virus infection. Virology. 2015;**479-480**:672-686. DOI: 10.1016/j.virol.2015.02.031

[60] Liao W, Ou JH. Phosphorylation and nuclear localization of the hepatitis B virus core protein: Significance of serine in the three repeated SPRRR motifs. Journal of Virology. 1995;**69**:1025-1029

[61] Ning X, Basagoudanavar SH, Liu K, Luckenbaugh L, Wei D, Wang C, et al. Capsid phosphorylation state and hepadnavirus virion secretion. Journal of Virology. 2017;**91**:1-16. DOI: 10.1128/jvi.00092-17

[62] Zhao Q, Hu Z, Cheng J, Wu S, Luo Y, Chang J, et al. Hepatitis B virus core protein dephosphorylation occurs during pregenomic RNA encapsidation. Journal of Virology. 2018;**92**:1-18. DOI: 10.1128/jvi.02139-17

[63] Bottcher B, Vogel M, Ploss M, Nassal M. High plasticity of the hepatitis B virus capsid revealed by conformational stress. Journal of Molecular Biology. 2006;**356**:812-822. DOI: 10.1016/j.jmb.2005.11.053

[64] Meng D, Hjelm RP, Hu J, Wu J. A theoretical model for the dynamic

structure of hepatitis B nucleocapsid. Biophysical Journal. 2011;**101**:2476-2484. DOI: 10.1016/j.bpj.2011.10.002

[65] Roseman AM, Berriman JA, Wynne SA, Butler PJ, Crowther RA. A structural model for maturation of the hepatitis B virus core. Proceedings of the National Academy of Sciences of the United States of America. 2005;**102**:15821-15826. DOI: 10.1073/pnas.0504874102

[66] Lewellyn EB, Loeb DD. The arginine clusters of the carboxy-terminal domain of the core protein of hepatitis B virus make pleiotropic contributions to genome replication. Journal of Virology. 2011;**85**:1298-1309. DOI: 10.1128/JVI.01957-10

[67] Schmitz A, Schwarz A, Foss M, Zhou L, Rabe B, Hoellenriegel J, et al. Nucleoporin 153 arrests the nuclear import of hepatitis B virus capsids in the nuclear basket. PLoS Pathogens. 2010;**6**:e1000741. DOI: 10.1371/journal.ppat.1000741

[68] Blondot ML, Bruss V, Kann M. Intracellular transport and egress of hepatitis B virus. Journal of Hepatology. 2016;**64**:S49-S59. DOI: 10.1016/j.jhep.2016.02.008

[69] Summers J, Mason WS. Replication of the genome of a hepatitis B-like virus by reverse transcription of an RNA intermediate. Cell. 1982;**29**:403-415. DOI: 10.1016/0092-8674(82)90157-x

[70] Ning X, Luckenbaugh L, Liu K, Bruss V, Sureau C, Hu J. Common and distinct capsid and surface protein requirements for secretion of complete and genome-free hepatitis B virions. Journal of Virology. 2018;**92**:1-18. DOI: 10.1128/jvi.00272-18

[71] Ning X, Nguyen D, Mentzer L, Adams C, Lee H, Ashley R, et al. Secretion of genome-free hepatitis B virus—Single strand blocking model for virion morphogenesis of para-retrovirus. PLoS Pathogens. 2011;**7**:e1002255. DOI: 10.1371/journal.ppat.1002255

[72] Liu K, Hu J. Secretion of empty or complete hepatitis B virions: Envelopment of empty capsids versus mature nucleocapsids. Future Virology. 2019;**14**:95-105. DOI: 10.2217/fvl-2018-0128

[73] Bottcher B, Nassal M. Structure of mutant hepatitis B core protein capsids with premature secretion phenotype. Journal of Molecular Biology. 2018;**430**:4941-4954. DOI: 10.1016/j.jmb.2018.10.018

[74] Pastor F, Herrscher C, Patient R, Moreau A, Burlaud-Gaillard J, Seigneuret F, et al. Direct interaction between hepatitis B virus core and envelope proteins analyzed in a cellular context. Scientific Reports. 7 November 2019;**9**(1):16178-16190. DOI: 10.1038/s41598-019-52824-z

[75] Ponsel D, Bruss V. Mapping of amino acid side chains on the surface of hepatitis B virus capsids required for envelopment and virion formation. Journal of Virology. 2003;**77**:416-422

[76] Yuan TT, Sahu GK, Whitehead WE, Greenberg R, Shih C. The mechanism of an immature secretion phenotype of a highly frequent naturally occurring missense mutation at codon 97 of human hepatitis B virus core antigen. Journal of Virology. 1999;**73**:5731-5740

[77] Martinez MG, Testoni B, Zoulim F. Biological basis for functional cure of chronic hepatitis B. Journal of Viral Hepatitis. 2019;**26**:786-794. DOI: 10.1111/jvh.13090

[78] Testoni B, Durantel D, Zoulim F. Novel targets for hepatitis B virus therapy. Liver International: Official Journal of the International Association for the Study of the Liver. 2017;**37**(Suppl 1):33-39. DOI: 10.1111/liv.13307

[79] Wang JC, Dhason MS, Zlotnick A. Structural organization of pregenomic RNA and the carboxy-terminal domain of the capsid protein of hepatitis B virus. PLoS Pathogens. 2012;**8**:e1002919. DOI: 10.1371/journal.ppat.1002919

[80] Olson ED, Musier-Forsyth K. Retroviral Gag protein-RNA interactions: Implications for specific genomic RNA packaging and virion assembly. Seminars in Cell and Developmental Biology. 2019;**86**:129-139. DOI: 10.1016/j.semcdb.2018.03.015

[81] Rein A, Datta SA, Jones CP, Musier-Forsyth K. Diverse interactions of retroviral Gag proteins with RNAs. Trends in Biochemical Sciences. 2011;**36**:373-380. DOI: 10.1016/j.tibs.2011.04.001

[82] Gatignol A. Transcription of HIV: Tat and cellular chromatin. Advances in Pharmacology (San Diego, Calif.). 2007;**55**:137-159. DOI: 10.1016/s1054-3589(07)55004-0

[83] Karn J. The molecular biology of HIV latency: Breaking and restoring the Tat-dependent transcriptional circuit. Current Opinion in HIV and AIDS. 2011;**6**:4-11. DOI: 10.1097/COH.0b013e328340ffbb

[84] Lott L, Notvall L, Lanford RE. Transcomplementation of core and polymerase functions of the woolly monkey and human hepatitis B viruses. Virology. 2003;**308**:330-339. DOI: 10.1016/s0042-6822(03)00003-5

[85] Protzer U, Nassal M, Chiang P-W, Kirschfink M, Schaller H. Interferon gene transfer by a hepatitis B virus vector efficiently suppresses wild-type virus infection. Proceedings of the National Academy of Sciences. 1999;**96**:10818. DOI: 10.1073/pnas.96.19.10818

[86] Ludgate L, Liu K, Luckenbaugh L, Streck N, Eng S, Voitenleitner C, et al. Cell-free hepatitis B virus capsid assembly dependent on the core protein C-terminal domain and regulated by phosphorylation. Journal of Virology. 2016;**90**:5830-5844. DOI: 10.1128/JVI.00394-16

[87] Newman M, Chua PK, Tang FM, Su PY, Shih C. Testing an electrostatic interaction hypothesis of hepatitis B virus capsid stability by using an in vitro capsid disassembly/reassembly system. Journal of Virology. 2009;**83**:10616-10626. DOI: 10.1128/jvi.00749-09

[88] Gallina A, Bonelli F, Zentilin L, Rindi G, Muttini M, Milanesi G. A recombinant hepatitis B core antigen polypeptide with the protamine-like domain deleted self-assembles into capsid particles but fails to bind nucleic acids. Journal of Virology. 1989;**63**:4645-4652

[89] Gazina EV, Fielding JE, Lin B, Anderson DA. Core protein phosphorylation modulates pregenomic RNA encapsidation to different extents in human and duck hepatitis B viruses. Journal of Virology. 2000;**74**:4721-4728

[90] Kann M, Sodeik B, Vlachou A, Gerlich WH, Helenius A. Phosphorylation-dependent binding of hepatitis B virus core particles to the nuclear pore complex. The Journal of Cell Biology. 1999;**145**:45-55

[91] Yu X, Jin L, Jih J, Shih C, Zhou ZH. 3.5A cryoEM structure of hepatitis B virus core assembled from full-length core protein. PLoS ONE. 2013;**8**:e69729. DOI: 10.1371/journal.pone.0069729

[92] Nair S, Zlotnick A. Asymmetric modification of hepatitis B virus (HBV) genomes by an endogenous cytidine deaminase inside HBV cores informs a model of reverse transcription. Journal of Virology. 2018;**92**:15261-15269. DOI: 10.1128/jvi.02190-17

[93] Liu G, Ma X, Wang Z, Wakae K, Yuan Y, He Z, et al. Adenosine

deaminase acting on RNA-1 (ADAR1) inhibits hepatitis B virus (HBV) replication by enhancing microRNA-122 processing. The Journal of Biological Chemistry. 2019;**294**:14043-14054. DOI: 10.1074/jbc.RA119.007970

[94] Chen Y, Hu J, Cai X, Huang Y, Zhou X, Tu Z, et al. APOBEC3B edits HBV DNA and inhibits HBV replication during reverse transcription. Antiviral Research. 2018;**149**:16-25. DOI: 10.1016/j.antiviral.2017.11.006

[95] Cuevas JM, Geller R, Garijo R, Lopez-Aldeguer J, Sanjuan R. Extremely high mutation rate of HIV-1 in vivo. PLoS Biology. 2015;**13**:e1002251. DOI: 10.1371/journal.pbio.1002251

[96] Huang ZS, Su WH, Wang JL, Wu HN. Selective strand annealing and selective strand exchange promoted by the N-terminal domain of hepatitis delta antigen. The Journal of Biological Chemistry. 2003;**278**:5685-5693. DOI: 10.1074/jbc.M207938200

[97] Huang ZS, Wu HN. Identification and characterization of the RNA chaperone activity of hepatitis delta antigen peptides. The Journal of Biological Chemistry. 1998;**273**:26455-26461. DOI: 10.1074/jbc.273.41.26455

[98] Ivanyi-Nagy R, Kanevsky I, Gabus C, Lavergne JP, Ficheux D, Penin F, et al. Analysis of hepatitis C virus RNA dimerization and core-RNA interactions. Nucleic Acids Research. 2006;**34**:2618-2633

[99] Mir MA, Panganiban AT. Characterization of the RNA chaperone activity of hantavirus nucleocapsid protein. Journal of Virology. 2006;**80**:6276-6285. DOI: 10.1128/jvi.00147-06

[100] Pong WL, Huang ZS, Teoh PG, Wang CC, Wu HN. RNA binding property and RNA chaperone activity of dengue virus core protein and other viral RNA-interacting proteins. FEBS Letters. 2011;**585**:2575-2581. DOI: 10.1016/j.febslet.2011.06.038

[101] Wang SH, Syu WJ, Huang KJ, Lei HY, Yao CW, King CC, et al. Intracellular localization and determination of a nuclear localization signal of the core protein of dengue virus. The Journal of General Virology. 2002;**83**:3093-3102. DOI: 10.1099/0022-1317-83-12-3093

[102] Xu X, Severson W, Villegas N, Schmaljohn CS, Jonsson CB. The RNA binding domain of the hantaan virus N protein maps to a central, conserved region. Journal of Virology. 2002;**76**:3301-3308. DOI: 10.1128/jvi.76.7.3301-3308.2002

[103] Zuniga S, Sola I, Moreno JL, Sabella P, Plana-Duran J, Enjuanes L. Coronavirus nucleocapsid protein is an RNA chaperone. Virology. 2007;**357**:215-227. DOI: 10.1016/j.virol.2006.07.046

[104] Rumnieks J, Tars K. Protein-RNA interactions in the single-stranded RNA bacteriophages. Sub-Cellular Biochemistry. 2018;**88**:281-303. DOI: 10.1007/978-981-10-8456-0_13

[105] Kulkarni P, Uversky VN. Intrinsically disordered proteins and the Janus challenge. Biomolecules. 2018;**8**. DOI: 10.3390/biom8040179

[106] Takeshita D, Tomita K. Assembly of Q[beta] viral RNA polymerase with host translational elongation factors EF-Tu and -Ts. Proceedings of the National Academy of Sciences of the United States of America. 2010;**107**:15733-15738. DOI: 10.1073/pnas.1006559107

Chapter 2

E1 and E2 Viral Proteins as Therapeutic Targets for Development of Antiviral Agents

María Leticia Saucedo-Mendiola, José Luis Ríos-Bañuelos, Alejandra Vázquez-Vázquez, Elva Marcela Coria-Quiñones, María Estela Frías-Zepeda, Jesús Alonso Gándara-Mireles and Adolfo Padilla-Mendiola

Abstract

The importance of studying the human papillomavirus (HPV) is because it is a disease that relies on 14 HPV types classified as carcinogenic high risk and that contributes to cervical cancers affecting approximately 527,600 women yearly and causing 265,387 deaths yearly, being the second mortality cause for women globally. In Mexico, 13.9% of demises are due to cervical uterine cancer (CUCA). The challenges for a vaccine that may prevent HPV occurrence are an active field for scientists with significant advances but still undergoing for a full cure to this disease. In this work, latest research trends to treat HPV are analyzed, and by means of molecular coupling analysis, a modeling and simulation process to predict interactions of leader molecules with the target for synthetic elaboration of a possible therapeutic treatment is developed. One of the main topics discussed in this chapter relates to new drug design for HPV treatment, which is related to the inhibitors of protein-protein interactions and in the protein drugs. Regarding HPV therapy development, a group of small molecules has been identified using high-performance sieving capable of interrupting HPV16 E1-E2 interaction, which helps avoid viral replication. Some of these compounds displayed nanomolar affinities and high specificity.

Keywords: viral proteins, human papillomavirus, HPV, E1-E2 proteins, TDDFT

1. Introduction

Human papillomavirus (HPV) belongs to the Papillomaviridae family, according to the eighth report developed by the International Committee for Viral Taxonomy. To date, over 100 different HPV types have been cataloged and around 30 infected anogenital mucosae. HPV types are classified as virus from low to high risk according to their capability to cause benign or carcinogenic injuries, respectively [1].

Infection provoked by HPV is one of the more common causes among sexually transmitted diseases with prevalence levels varying between the population and geographic location.

IntechOpen

At least 14 types of them are classified as carcinogenic high risk (hr-HPV); among them HPV16 and HPV18 are responsible for around 70% of all cervical cancers affecting approximately 527,600 women yearly and causing 265,387 deaths yearly, being the second mortality cause for women globally [2]. Over 85% of new cases and deaths referred occur in developing countries [3] such as Mexico, where 13.9% of demises are due to cervical uterine cancer (CUCA) [4].

The challenges for a vaccine that may prevent HPV occurrence is an active field for scientists with significant advances but still undergoing for a full solution that can eliminate this disease.

In this work latest research trends to treat HPV are analyzed, and by means of molecular coupling analysis, a modeling and simulation process to predict interactions of leader molecules with the target for synthetic elaboration of a possible therapeutic treatment is developed.

This chapter is a review of the latest advances on new drug design for HPV treatment which are related to the inhibitors of protein-protein interactions and in the protein drugs. Regarding HPV therapy development, a group of small molecules has been identified using high -performance sieving capable of interrupting HPV16 E1-E2 interaction which helps avoid viral replication. Some of these compounds displayed nanomolar affinities and high specificity.

2. HPV genome, treatment, and prevention

2.1 HPV infection, treatment, and prevention

Currently, an antiviral treatment is unavailable that can help eliminate the infection or avoid progression of injuries caused by CUCA. Current therapies for cervical dysplasia and cancer implicate destruction or elimination of infected tissue by cytotoxic agents or surgery [5]. On the other hand, FDA has approved three vaccines for HPV infection prevention: Gardasil, Gardasil 9, and Cervarix. All three prevent HPV infection types 16 and 18 [6, 7]. Gardasil also protects HPV infection types 6 and 11, which cause 90% of genital warts [8]. Gardasil 9 protects from infection of the same four HPV types and other five HPV types (31/33/45/52/58) that cause cancer [9]. These vaccines are based in empty particles similar to the "ghost" virus, formed by L1 protein capsid from each viral type [8, 10]. It has been demonstrated that these vaccines are highly protective against the lesions of transformed cells at an early stage that represent cervical cancer precursors. Since HPV 16 and HPV 18 currently represent the two HR-HPV more common in most geographical locations, universal adoption of the vaccines may protect more than two-thirds of HPV-induced cancers [10].

However, vaccination programs are not implemented worldwide, and coverage is still very low especially in low-income countries [10, 11].

It has been estimated that the addition of HPV 31/33/45/52/58 to the nine-valent vaccine could prevent almost 90% of cases of invasive cervical cancer worldwide [12, 13].

HPV vaccines currently available are useful tools in the fight against HPV infections and cancers but provide an incomplete answer for long-term HPV disease eradication. By their very nature of being capable of inducing a strong and protective humural—but no cellular—host immune response, they are also of little therapeutic value to already infected patients [10].

Scientists are working in new HPV therapeutic vaccines which may help avoid cancer formation in women previously infected with HPV [14]. These vaccines work by stimulating the immune system to attack and destroy infected cells. Clinical studies under development are evaluating safety and efficiency of a DNA therapeutic vaccine to treat injuries by HPV in the cervix and vulva. An ideal strategy would be to combine a preventive and a therapeutic vaccine. Another prevention strategy under testing is using external microbicidal. It has been found that carrageenan, a compound that can be extracted from seaweeds and extensively used in foods and other products, inhibits HPV infection in laboratory studies. A clinical study is under development to demonstrate if a gel containing carrageenan is capable to prevent genital infection by HPV in healthy individuals [15–17].

2.2 HPV genome

HPV genome (**Figure 1**) consists of a circular double-chain DNA molecule of approximately 8 Kb in size. The genome is organized in three regions. The region early contains the genes E1–E8 that code predominately for regulatory proteins essential for viral transcription and replication, as well as cell cycle control; the late region encodes for the two viral structural proteins, L1 and L2, needed for capsid formation and the noncoding region also known are long control region (LCR) or upstream regulatory region (URR). The LCR region varies in size between 800 and 1000 pb for the different HPV types, does no encodes any protein but, contains Cis-elements required for regulation of genes expression and genome replication [18].

2.3 HPV life cycle

HPV life cycle is coupled to the differentiation cell program experienced by epithelium keratinocytes. PVs are highly specific from the species they infect and present a tropism defined by epithelial scaly cells infecting undifferentiated basal cells.

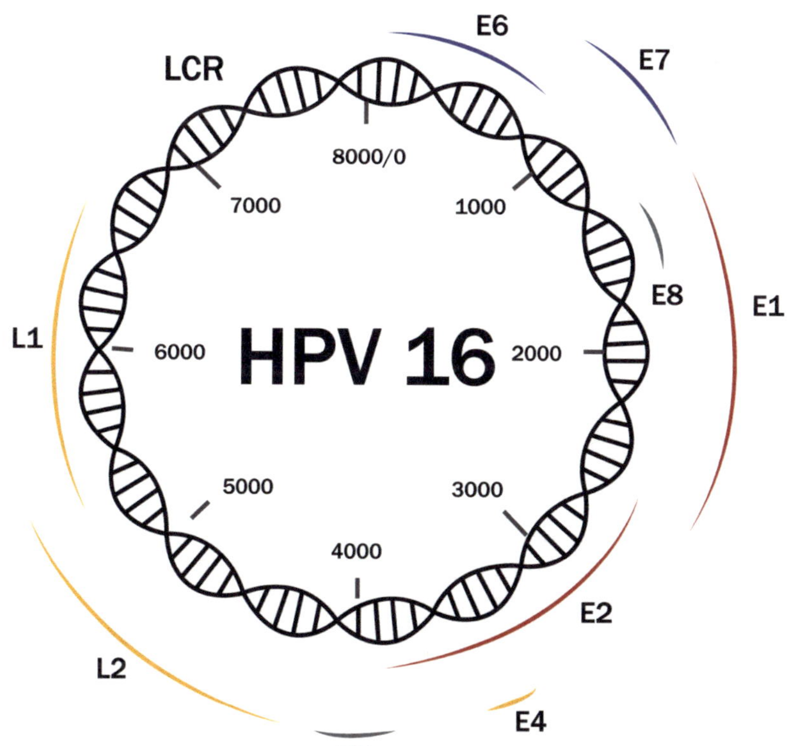

Figure 1.
Representation of HPV genome organization in a circular chain displaying the DNA molecule. LCR is the region noncoding the open reading frames (ORFs) encode the early (E) and late (L) viral proteins [18].

During epithelium mucosa infection, firs of all, virions need to reach the undifferentiated basal cells. Once in contact with blank cells, virion is associated with putative receptors such as alpha integrins, heparins, and laminins probably through wounds or microabrasions that give access to basal zones at the epithelium [19].

Heparin sulfate proteoglycans (HSPGs) from the cellular surface seem to be the primary receptor for initial binding [20]. The joint together is mediated by the last 15 amino acids from the extreme carboxyl-terminal of L1 protein [21]. Virions enter the cell by endocytosis by using the clathrin-dependent route. Decapsidation of the particle occurs at the endosome, releasing the capsid genome and proteins in the endocytic vesicles [22].

After HPV infects basal cells, viral genome is established as a multiple copies episome at the cells' nuclei through several viral DNA replication cycles.

Conservation of the viral episome at 50–100 copies at these undifferentiated cells is obtained then through low DNA replication levels, and it is essential for the infection persistence; by itself it is a risk factor for carcinogenesis induced by the virus; the first proteins to express themselves are the viral replication proteins E1 and E2. E2 protein presents a characteristic regulating function affecting the transcription, the replication, and the episome conservation [20, 23].

During the productive infection, viral protein detection at the basal layers barely exists, even though E7 protein may be detected by cervical neoplasia, where the expression levels cannot be controlled properly [23]. Proliferative basal cells would migrate to parabasal and intermediate layers, starting the differentiation program and with it the transcription of the different early viral genes, regulated through the LCR region. During this period DNA will replicate hundreds of copies by cell, thanks to E6 and E7 proteins which will block the exit of cells from the cellular cycle [24].

During productive infection, HPV proteins cannot easily be detected in the basal cell layer, although the E7 protein can be seen in cervical neoplasia where expression levels are not properly controlled.

As HPV-infected cells divide and differentiate, the late HPV promoter is activated mediated by transcription factors dependent on the differentiation, this has as consequence the amplification of the viral DNA, and an increase in the levels of viral proteins needed for replication, including E1, E4 and E5, being E4 the more abundant.

It has been suggested that E7 continuous expression in a cell containing abundant E4 which favors the conservation of the cell in phase S, this allows the viral genome accumulation.

When basal cells enter the differentiation process that will convert them into keratinocytes, at the same time they migrate to superior layers in the epithelium that will cause an explosion in the viral DNA replication, known as vegetative replication.

Finally, both proteins and the capsid (L1 and L2) are expressed only in cells that have passed through the vegetative viral amplification. At the end of the productive cycle, genomes will encapsidate, generating virions that will be let out with release of superior layer cells from the mucous epithelium [23].

HPV DNA replication initiates with the cooperative join of E1 and E2 with specific DNA sequences inside the viral origin [15–17]. Formation of this ternary compound E1-E2-ori depends on the interaction between both proteins with DNA, but also there is a critical interaction between the E2 transactivation domain of N-terminal (TAD) and the E1 enzymatic domain of E1 C-terminal [25]. Assembly of this initial complex E1-E2-ori is the starting point for additional E1 molecule recruitment [26, 27] and its assembly in hexamers and double hexamers that display activity in ATPase and helicase [28, 29]. Any of the protein–protein and protein-DNA interactions produced in the origin could be directed toward the development of small antiviral molecules to treat infections by HPV.

It has been demonstrated clearly that expression E1 and E2 proteins from different HPV genomes can induce replication of the genomic integrated HPV origin [30], and this is a particular danger in the presence of DNA damage [31]. Then, anti-HPV agents unblocking viral DNA synthesis could, in time, benefit cancer development increasing HPV genome integration. Due to E1 and E2 capability to induce HPV DNA integration, HPV DNA replication through E1 interactions with cellular replication proteins probably may represent one of the best approaches to develop an HPV antiviral that also prevents HPV integration at the host cell chromosomes.

2.4 E1 and E2 proteins as therapeutic targets

E1 is the most conserved protein among the papillomavirus and the only with enzymatic activity [32, 33]. This situation adds up to the fact that viral DNA replication is absolutely dependent on E1, and it has contributed to do an attractive target out of this protein so antiviral agents may be developed.

E1 gene is the bigger and one of the more conserved PVs with approximately 2 Kb, and it codifies E1 multimeric protein [28].

E1 protein has three functional domains. C-terminal domain has helicase/ATPase, and it participates in viral DNA replication and includes sequences involved in the protein oligomerization [34, 35].

Variable length central region contains the DNA-binding domain (DBD), which recognizes specific sites at the ori but with low affinity [36–38], and an N-terminal regulator region which is essential for live optimal replication [39, 40].

The last one codifies several functional elements, such as a nuclear localization sequence (NLS), a nuclear export sequence (NES), a joint cyclin motif, and Cdk2 phosphorylation sites. E1 N-terminal regulator region for HPV anogenital type also interact with cellular p80 protein known alternatively as UAF1 or WDR48 [41].

Terminal carboxyl domain and spacer region have been widely studied. However, N-terminal domain functions have not been well defined other than those related to the nuclear location [35].

DBD of E1 protein consists in a sequence of 60 pb approximately. This sequence contains three elements, a sequence rich in A and T, a palindrome sequence found at LCR, forming hexamers and double hexamer, and a 12 pb sequence that constitutes a joining site for E2 protein [42, 43].

DBD has been widely characterized in vitro and it was the first E1 domain to be crystallized [43–45]. And this reveals an unusual joint mode to DNA by an extended bond and an α helix forming a continuous surface as DNA join.

Even though DBD more important function is to recognize and mark the ori, it has other functions as well. DBD performs an important role in the fusion of bicatenary DNA and the formation of hexameric replicative helicase [43].

The E1 N-terminal region is formed by 200 amino acids approximately; it is the less preserved segment of this protein. This region contains a number of motifs from short sequence amino acids preserved as variable among different PVs, including a nuclear localization signal (NLS), a nuclear export signal of dependent-Crm1 (NES), and a joining motif to the cyclin (CBM) that interacts with cyclin A/E in complex with kinase dependent of cyclin 2 (Cdk2) and Cdk2 phosphorylation sites and other kinases [40, 46, 47].

The E2 gene has approximately 1100 bp codifies a nuclear protein of 45 kDa [18, 48], E2 protein is composed of three functional domains. The first, at

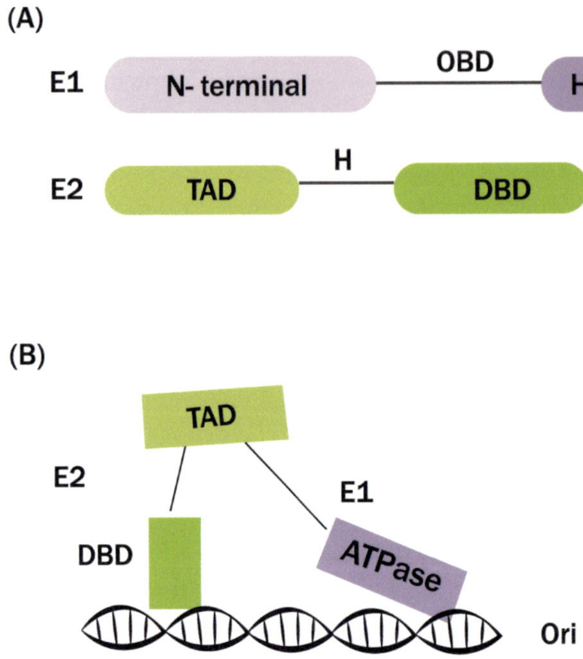

Figure 2.
Initiation of HPV DNA replication. (A) Schematic representation of the viral proteins E1 and E2 required for replication of the HPV genome. E1 and E2 are approximately 650 and 370 amino acids in length, respectively. Locations of the different functional domains in each protein are indicated. OBD, origin binding domain helicase/ATPase N-terminal; TAD, transactivation domain; H, hinge region; DBD, DNA-binding domain. (B) Schematic diagram of the initiation of HPV DNA replication. (I) Replication is initiated by the recruitment of E1 (purple) and by E2 (green), to the viral origin [10].

the extreme amino terminal, is the activation domain (E2TAD), responsible of regulating the transcription and replication of the viral genome [18, 48]. The second domain is a hinge or central domain, with more variable length and sequence among the HPVs. The third domain at the carboxyl-terminal is for dimerization and binding with the DNA, and it is formed by 100 amino acids approximately [18, 48, 49]. Crystal structure E2 protein from all viral strains have in common the fact of joining a palindromic DNA sequence (ACCgNNNNcGGT, lower case letters indicate preferred nucleotides; NNNN region is called spacing region), referred as the E2 union site. Nevertheless, there are specific differences in viral strains in regard to E2 protein ability to discriminate union sites [48] (**Figure 2**).

HPV protein E2 displays independent complex functions regarding the transcription and may be able to modulate host cells with respect to the viral replication cycle [48–50].

3. Computational modeling of E1 and E2 inhibitors

Several pharmaceutical companies have invested resources in the identification of E1 ATPase/helicase inhibitors. Even though small molecules have been identified as capable to inhibit this enzyme activity, unfortunately, none of these projects has resulted in a viable therapy. In late years, antiviral research has begun to deal with the vital interactions modulation between proteins and proteins as a feasible therapeutic way.

An interaction protein–protein essential in the HPV DNA replication is the interaction between HPV E1 and E2 proteins. There are diverse reported works with advances in identification of leader compounds that may interrupt protein–protein E1-E2 interactions. Some of these compounds showed nanomolar affinities and high specificity.

Yoakim and coworker [51] discovered a group of small molecules known as indanones, and this molecules showed the capability to inhibit specifically E1-E2 protein interaction, which also have been identified as the first inhibitors for small molecules capable to antagonize the assembly of E1-E2 complex and the viral ori HPV11. It was identified a compound that inhibited E1-E2 protein interaction by means of high-performance sieving from the collection of over Boehringer Ingelheim 100,000 compounds, using a scintillation proximity assay (SPA). Also, more active analogues were synthesized that were capable to inhibit the E1-E2 complex assembly with the HPV11 viral ori with low nanomolar power in vitro and with activity in cell culture. Structurally, this group of inhibitors presents an indandione system spirofused onto a substituted tetrahydrofuran ring which were denominated as indandione inhibitors. It was determined that these inhibitors act by joining to E2 TAD domain, the same protein region that interacts with E1 [51, 52]. Crystalline structures, HPV11 E2 TAD by itself or as a complex with an indandione inhibitor, both provide a detailed comprehension of the mechanism in which indandione inhibitors join E2 to interrupt the interaction E1-E2. A comparison between both structures revealed that the union between the inhibitors caused insignificant alterations on the protein backbone, but it did induce a significant movement of several lateral amino acid chains at the union site. These changes in the lateral chain conformation, particularly from Tyr-19, His-32, Leu-94 y, and Glu-100 residues, resulted in the formation of a deep hydrophobic bag that is joined firmly to the inhibitor indandione fraction. The structure also revealed that the inhibitor carboxylate fraction, known by its importance for power, forms hydrogen bonds with amides from the protein backbone. Studies regarding the structure-activity relationship (SAR) revealed that the carboxylate fraction is important in potency of the inhibitor. Mechanistic studies, including the use of isothermal titling calorimetry, showed that the indandione inhibitors join reversibly to E2 TAD with 1:1 stoichiometry. Even though indandione inhibitors displayed a powerful activity against E2 proteins of low-risk viruses HPV6 and HPV11, these did not show any activity against high-risk types HPV16, HPV18, and HPV31. Cellular culture studies showed that indandione inhibitors are capable of antagonizing E1-E2 interaction of HPV6 and HPV11 [49].

3.1 Other labs' approach

White and coworker addressed these issues in a series of detailed studies to identify inhibitors of the cooperative assembly of HPV E1 and E2 on the ori, focusing on HPV 6 and 11. They identified two series of inhibitors that bound to overlapping sites at the E1 binding interface on the E2 TAD. Results obtained from modeling works suggest that inhibitors derived from repaglinide form weak interactions with protein E2 TAD but occupy a bigger portion from the inhibitor union bag than the indandione series.

Both series of compounds were optimized for binding by medicinal chemistry approaches, and in both series the best compounds in each series had low nanomolar activity against the HPV 11 E1-E2 interaction.

The fact that the potent repaglinide derivatives, with values IC_{50} at nanomolar range against HPV6 and HPV11 E2, and EC_{50} values in cellular DNA replication assays of approximately 1 mM, make this series a promising route for development of small molecular inhibitors for E1-E2 interaction [53].

Capabilities of indandione compounds to inhibit HPV genome in vivo replication, especially low-risk HPV types, demonstrate for the first time the therapeutic potential of protein E2 as target for the development of small molecule inhibitors at HPV protein interaction, particularly in the case for treatment of anogenital warts caused by HPV6 and HPV11. Furthermore, location and characterization of the union bag for E2 TAD inhibitors provide a new potential therapeutic option for treatment of HPV infections. These studies have set the basis for the use of approaches based in structures for rational design or for virtual selection of inhibitor compounds capable of joining to all or part of the identified inhibitor union bag.

Kantang and coworker worked in the prediction of the interactions of the helicase domain of the E1 protein of HPV16 and the TAD domain of HPV16; for this purpose, E1 protein domain was modeled (residue 421–622) from HPV16 with I-TASSER server. The model with the best C-score was selected to coupling to structure E2 from HPV16 and HPV18 using ClusPro. Superposition of E1 HPV16 and the crystalline structure of E1 HPV18 showed an RMSD of 1.39 Å, indicating structural similitude. A complex structure for HPV16 E1-E2 is also predicted as similar to crystalline structure of HPV18 E1-E2, with an RMSD value of 1.11 Å. An analysis of HPV16 E1-E2 interactions revealed there are three sites for interaction of complex HPV16 E1 and E2. The residues Glu118, and Tyr178 at the structural domain of folded β-sheet for HPV16 E2 form hydrogen bonds with Tyr578, Arg575, Ser574, Asp573 of HPV16 E1, respectively.

HPV16 E2 helicoidal N-terminal domain is the main union site for HPV16 E1 protein where Asp13, Thr17, Tyr19, Asp22, Tyr32, Glu39, and Val58 from HPV16 E2 interact with Arg615 (for Asp13 and Thr17 E2), Arg447, Arg619, Glu452, Arg447, and Tyr602 from HPV16 E1, respectively. Shows Gln95 and Glu100; at the linking segment between N-terminal and C-terminal HPV16 E2, there are interactions with Arg462 and Ser455 from HPV16 E1, respectively. Besides, structures of nine peptides reported [54] were built by I-TASSER server. Using ClusPro web server, it was able to predict binding, conformations, and interactions of peptides with HPV16 E2 protein; bind conformations and interactions between small peptides and HPV16 E2 protein were predicted and analyzed. These results were used ahead for the design of more powerful peptides that may potentially inhibit E1-E2 complex formation. Binding affinities obtained for designed peptides and protein E2 of HPV16 recombinant were in good agreement with experimental results. Four peptides were the more efficient inhibitors of E1-E2 complex, and they could be used for suppression of HPV replication [55].

4. Conclusions

Currently a cure or treatment for HPV is unavailable. In many men and women, HPV disappears by itself without causing further problems. There are treatments for affections caused by the virus. Among these affections are genital warts, precarcinogenic cells, and cancer.

Even though there are vaccines against the main HPV types, there are therapeutic treatments needed for those that have been already exposed to the virus which represent most of the population affected by this disease. In this regard, a diversity of research work related to antiviral design exists, including those work using computational methods. These studies have laid the foundation for the use of structure-based approaches to rationally design or virtually screen inhibitory compounds that are capable of preventing HPV replication.

By means of molecular coupling analysis, it is possible to predict interactions of leader molecules with the target with enough detail to be useful for synthetic elaboration of those molecules.

It has been considered that protein-protein interactions are difficult to inhibit because they often involve big surfaces, depriving small molecules to bind with the pocket; however, they are receiving great attention to work as targets for the rational design of drugs. The interest in the protein-protein interaction inhibitors and in the protein drugs has been in constant growth.

Regarding HPV therapy development, a group of small molecules has been identified using high-performance sieving capable of interrupting HPV16 E1-E2 interaction which helps avoid viral replication.

Acknowledgements

We thank the Scientific Computational Laboratory at FCQ-UJED for the computational resources and also MBA Fátima Berenice Corrales Saucedo for her contribution with graphic design.

Conflict of interest

The authors state that this research was completed without any conflicts of interest related with the funding to develop the present work.

Author details

María Leticia Saucedo-Mendiola[1*], José Luis Ríos-Bañuelos[1], Alejandra Vázquez-Vázquez[1], Elva Marcela Coria-Quiñones[1], María Estela Frías-Zepeda[1,2], Jesús Alonso Gándara-Mireles[2] and Adolfo Padilla-Mendiola[1]

1 Faculty of Chemistry Science, Juarez University of Durango State, Durango, México

2 CIIDIR-IPN, Durango, México

*Address all correspondence to: sauced101@yahoo.com.mx

References

[1] Bernard HU, Burk RD, Chen Z, van Doorslaer K, zur Hausen H, de Villiers EM. Classification of papillomaviruses (PVs) based on 189 PV types and proposal of taxonomic amendments. Virology. 2010;**401**(1):70-79

[2] World Health Organization (WHO). Available from: https://www.who.int/. [Accessed: 05 February 2018]

[3] Sánchez-Barriga JJ. Tendencias de mortalidad por cáncer cervicouterino en las siete regiones socioeconómicas y en las 32 entidades federativas de México en los años 2000-2008. Gaceta Médica de México. 2012;**148**:42-51

[4] Secretaría de Salud, México. 2014. Available from: http://www.sinais.salud.gob.mx

[5] Carrillo A, Hernández M, Hernández T, Zárate A. Terapéutica en infección de virus del papiloma humano. Articuló de revisión. Ginecología y Obstetricia de México. 2012;**80**(11):712-719

[6] Chaturvedi AK, Engels EA, Pfeiffer RM, et al. Human papillomavirus and rising oropharyngeal cancer incidence in the United States. Journal of Clinical Oncology. 2011;**29**(32):4294-4301

[7] Gillison ML, Chaturvedi AK, Lowy DR. HPV prophylactic vaccines and the potential prevention of noncervical cancers in both men and women. Cancer. 2008;**113**(10 Suppl):3036-3046

[8] Koutsky LA, Ault KA, Wheeler CM, et al. A controlled trial of a human papillomavirus type 16 vaccine. New England Journal of Medicine. 2002;**347**(21):1645-1651

[9] Trimble CL, Morrow MP, Kraynyak KA, et al. Safety, efficacy, and immunogenicity of VGX-3100, a therapeutic synthetic DNA vaccine targeting human papillomavirus 16 and 18 E6 and E7 proteins for cervical intraepithelial neoplasia 2/3: A randomised, double-blind, placebo-controlled phase 2b trial. Lancet. 2015;**386**(10008):2078-2088

[10] Archambault J, Melendy T. Targeting human papillomavirus genome replication for antiviral drug discovery. Antiviral Therapy. 2013;**18**(3):271-283

[11] Serrano B, Alemany L, Tous S, Bruni L, Clifford GM, Weiss T, et al. Potential impact of a nine-valent vaccine in human papillomavirus related cervical disease. Infectious Agents and Cancer. 2012;**7**(1):38

[12] Riethmuller D, Jacquard AC, Lacau St Guily J, Aubin F, Carcopino X, Pradat P, et al. Potential impact of a nonavalent HPV vaccine on the occurrence of HPV-related diseases in France. BMC Public Health. 2015;**15**:453

[13] Hartwig S, Baldauf JJ, Dominiak-Felden G, Simondon F, Alemany L, de Sanjosé S, et al. Estimation of the epidemiological burden of HPV-related anogenital cancers, precancerous lesions, and genital warts in women and men in Europe: Potential additional benefit of a nine-valent second generation HPV vaccine compared to first generation HPV vaccines. Papillomavirus Research. 2015;**1**:90-100

[14] Hancock G, Hellner K, Dorrell L. Therapeutic HPV vaccines. Best Practice and Research. Clinical Obstetrics and Gynaecology. 2018;**47**:59-72

[15] Gee J, Weinbaum C, Sukumaran L, Markowitz LE. Quadrivalent HPV vaccine safety review and safety

monitoring plans for nine-valent HPV vaccine in the United States. Human Vaccines and Immunotherapeutics. 2016;**12**(6):1406-1417

[16] Kreimer AR, Herrero R, Sampson JN, et al. Evidence for single-dose protection by the bivalent HPV vaccine—Review of the Costa Rica HPV vaccine trial and future research studies. Vaccine. 2018;**36**(32):4774-4782

[17] Safaeian M, Sampson JN, Pan Y, et al. Durability of protection afforded by fewer doses of the HPV16/18 vaccine: The CVT trial. Journal of the National Cancer Institute. 2018;**110**(2):205-212. DOI: 10.1093/jnci/djx158

[18] López-Saavedra A, Lizano SM. Cáncer cérvicouterino y el virus del papiloma humano: La historia que no termina. Cancerologia. 2006;**1**(1):31-55

[19] Acheson NH. Fundamentals of Molecular Virology. 1st ed. Winsconsin: John Wiley & Sons Inc; 2007. pp. 263-270

[20] Graham SV. The human papillomavirus replication cycle, and its links to cancer progression: A comprehensive review. Clinical Science. 2017;**131**:2201-2221. DOI: 10.1042/CS20160786

[21] Joyce JG, Tung JS, Przysiecki CT, Cook JC, Lehman ED, Sands JA, et al. The L1 major capsid protein of human papillomavirus type 11 recombinant virus-like particles interacts with heparin and cell-surface glycosaminoglycans on human keratinocytes. The Journal of Biological Chemistry. 1999;**274**(9):5810-5822

[22] Kamper N, Day PM, Nowak T, Selinka HC, Florin L, Bolscher J, et al. A membrane-destabilizing peptide in capsid protein L2 is required for egress of papillomavirus genomes from endosomes. Journal of Virology. 2006;**80**(2):759-768

[23] Doorbar J. Papillomavirus life cycle organization and biomarker selection. Disease Markers. 2007;**23**(4):297-313

[24] Veríssimo FJ, Galvão AJM, Allyrio T, de Medeiros FA. Biology and natural history of human papillomavirus infection. Open Access Journal of Clinical Trials. 2013;**5**:1-12

[25] Zou N, Liu JS, Kuo SR, Broker TR, Chow LT. The carboxyl-terminal region of the human papillomavirus type 16 E1 protein determines E2 protein specificity during DNA replication. Journal of Virology. 1998;**72**:3436-3441

[26] Lusky M, Hurwitz J, Seo YS. The bovine papillomavirus E2 protein modulates the assembly of but is not stably maintained in a replication-competent multimeric E1-replication origin complex. Proceedings of the National Academy of Sciences. 1994;**91**:8895-8899

[27] Sanders CM, Stenlund A. Recruitment and loading of the E1 initiator protein: An ATP-dependent process catalysed by a transcription factor. The EMBO Journal. 1998;**17**:7044-7055

[28] Fouts ET, Egelman EH, Botchan MR. Biochemical and electron microscopic image analysis of the hexameric E1 helicase. The Journal of Biological Chemistry. 1999;**274**(7):4447-4458

[29] Sedman J, Stenlund A. The papillomavirus E1 protein forms a DNA-dependent hexameric complex with ATPase and DNA helicase activities. Journal of Virology. 1998;**72**:6893-6897

[30] Kadaja M, Isok-Paas H, Laos T, Ustav E, Ustav M. Mechanism of genomic instability in cells infected with the high-risk human papillomaviruses. PLoS Pathogens. 2009;**5**(4):e1000397

[31] Tsakogiannis D, Gortsilas P, Kyriakopoulou Z, Ruether IG, Dimitriou TG, Orfanoudakis G, et al. Sites of disruption within E1 and E2 genes of HPV16 and association with cervical dysplasia. Journal of Medical Virology. 2015;**87**(11):1973-1980. DOI: 10.1002/jmv.24256

[32] Wilson VG, West M, Woytek K, Rangasamy D. Papillomavirus E1 proteins: Form, function, and features. Virus Genes. 2002;**24**(3):275-290

[33] Stenlund A. Initiation of DNA replication: Lessons from viral initiator proteins. Nature Reviews. Molecular Cell Biology. 2003;**4**(10):777-785

[34] Enemark EJ, Joshua-Tor L. Mechanism of DNA translocation in a replicative hexameric helicase. Nature. 2006;**442**(7100):270-275

[35] Schuck S, Ruse C, Stenlund A. CK2 phosphorylation inactivates DNA binding by the papillomavirus E1 and E2 proteins. Journal of Virology. 2013;**87**(13):7668-7679

[36] Stenlund A. E1 initiator DNA binding specificity is unmasked by selective inhibition of non-specific DNA binding. The EMBO Journal. 2003;**22**(4):954-963

[37] Titolo S, Brault K, Majewski J, White PW, Archambault J. Characterization of the minimal DNA binding domain of the human papillomavirus E1 helicase: Fluorescence anisotropy studies and characterization of a dimerization-defective mutant protein. Journal of Virology. 2003;**77**(9):5178-5191

[38] Titolo S, Pelletier A, Pulichino AM, Brault K, Wardrop E, White PW, et al. Identification of domains of the human papillomavirus type 11 E1 helicase involved in oligomerization and binding to the viral origin. Journal of Virology. 2000;**74**(16):7349-7361

[39] Morin G, Fradet-Turcotte A, Di Lello P, Bergeron-Labrecque F, Omichinski JG, Archambault J. A conserved amphipathic helix in the N-terminal regulatory region of the papillomavirus E1 helicase is required for efficient viral DNA replication. Journal of Virology. 2011;**85**(11):5287-5300

[40] Fradet-Turcotte A, Moody C, Laimins LA, Archambault J. Nuclear export of human papillomavirus type 31 E1 is regulated by Cdk2 phosphorylation and required for viral genome maintenance. Journal of Virology. 2010;**84**(22):11747-11760

[41] Côté-Martin A, Moody C, Fradet-Turcotte A, D'Abramo CM, Lehoux M, Joubert S, et al. Human papillomavirus E1 helicase interacts with the WD repeat protein p80 to promote maintenance of the viral genome in keratinocytes. Journal of Virology. 2008;**82**(3):1271-1283

[42] Chen G, Stenlund A. The E1 initiator recognizes multiple overlapping sites in the papillomavirus origin of DNA replication. Journal of Virology. 2001;**75**(1):292-302

[43] Enemark EJ, Chen G, Vaughn DE, Stenlund A, Joshua-Tor L. Crystal structure of the DNA binding domain of the replication initiation protein E1 from papillomavirus. Molecular Cell. 2000;**6**(1):149-158

[44] Auster AS, Joshua-Tor L. The DNA-binding domain of human papillomavirus type 18 E1. Crystal structure, dimerization, and DNA binding. The Journal of Biological Chemistry. 2004;**279**(5):3733-3742

[45] Enemark EJ, Stenlund A, Joshua-Tor L. Crystal structures of two intermediates in the assembly of the papillomavirus replication initiation complex. The EMBO Journal. 2002;**21**(6):1487-1496

[46] Deng W, Lin BY, Jin G, Wheeler CG, Ma T, Harper JW, et al. Cyclin/CDK regulates the nucleocytoplasmic localization of the human papillomavirus E1 DNA helicase. Journal of Virology. 2004;**78**(24):13954-13965

[47] Lentz MR, Stevens SM Jr, Raynes J, Elkhoury N. A phosphorylation map of the bovine papillomavirus E1 helicase. Virology Journal. 2006;**3**(1):13. DOI: 10.1186/1743-422X-3-13

[48] Beltrán-Lissabet JF. Aspectos generales sobre la estructura y función de las proteínas codificadas por el virus del Papiloma Humano. CENIC Ciencias Biologicas. 2014;**45**(2):108-118

[49] Wang Y, Coulombe R, Cameron DR, Thauvette L, Massariol MJ, Amon LM, et al. Crystal structure of the E2 transactivation domain of human papillomavirus type 11 bound to a protein interaction inhibitor. The Journal of Biological Chemistry. 2004;**279**(8):6976-6985

[50] Ekalaksananan T, Jungpol W, Prasitthimay C, Wongjampa W, Kongyingyoes B, Pientong C. Polymorphisms and functional analysis of the intact human papillomavirus16 E2 gene. Asian Pacific Journal of Cancer Prevention. 2014;**15**(23):10255-10262

[51] Yoakim C, Ogilvie WW, Goudreau N, Naud J, Haché B, O'Meara JA, et al. Discovery of the first series of inhibitors of human papillomavirus type 11: Inhibition of the assembly of the E1-E2-origin DNA complex. Bioorganic and Medicinal Chemistry Letters. 2003;**13**(15):2539-2541

[52] White PW, Titolo S, Brault K, Thauvette L, Pelletier A, Welchner E, et al. Inhibition of human papillomavirus DNA replication by small molecule antagonists of the E1-E2 protein interaction. The Journal of Biological Chemistry. 2003;**278**(29):26765-26772

[53] White PW, Faucher AM, Goudreau N. Small molecule inhibitors of the human papillomavirus E1-E2 interaction. Current Topics in Microbiology and Immunology. 2011;**348**:61-88

[54] Fujii T, Austin D, Guo D, Srimatkandada S, Wang T, Kubushiro K, et al. Peptides inhibitory for the transcriptional regulatory function of human papillomavirus E2. Clinical Cancer Research. 2003;**9**:5423-5428

[55] Kantang W, Chunsrivirot S, Muangsin N, Poovorawan Y, Krusong K. Design of peptides as inhibitors of human papillomavirus 16 transcriptional regulator E1-E2. Chemical Biology and Drug Design. 2016;**88**(4):475-484

Chapter 3

Basic Research and Clinical Examination of Tumor Virus

Tatsuaki Tsuruyama, Shuichiro Ogawa and Norishige Yamada

Abstract

Tumor viruses cause cancer; thus, extensive studies are being conducted on them. In this article, we will review the basic medical research on the current clinical genetic tests for tumor viruses such as human papilloma virus, hepatitis B virus, and T-cell leukemia virus. Recently, clinical genetic tests have been developed for quick diagnosis of the tumor virus infection. Additionally, we will review the mutagenesis of murine leukemia retrovirus. In particular, we will focus on the insertional mutagenesis. This will help in deciding the direction of future virus research by combining clinical and basic research.

Keywords: tumor virus, gene analysis, clinical examination, cancer diseases

1. Introduction

1.1 History of tumor virus research

Tumor virus research is an important subject to understand the molecular biology of tumor viruses and carcinogenesis. Dr. Katsusaburo Yamagiwa, a Japanese pathologist, is famous for the experiment in which coal tar was applied to rabbit ears to induce carcinogenesis in 1915. He was also a candidate for the Nobel Prize in Medicine. The following year, his student Dr. Akira Fujinami was appointed to study carcinogenesis in Germany for 4 years. After returning to Japan, in 1900, he became the first professor at the Department of Pathology, Kyoto Imperial University Medical College. In 1905, he started studying chicken tumors, and as early as 1910, he established a chicken breast tumor transplant system. He had suggested the possibility of carcinogenesis by filterable pathogens, which were later called Fujinami sarcoma virus (FSV). He is also well known for the discovery of Japan schistosomiasis.

Interestingly, in the same year, Peyton Rous, who was studying at the Rockefeller laboratory in the United States, also established the avian sarcoma transplant system. In 1966, Rous received the Nobel Prize in Physiology and Medicine for the discovery of carcinogenic viruses. Hanafusa et al. elucidated the FSV gene structure and identified the similarity with the Rous sarcoma virus gene structure [1]. Both FSV and Rous sarcoma virus belong to the same alpha-retrovirus. FSV has the oncogene v-fps in its genome [2]. It also has long terminal repeats (LTRs) at the ends of the genome that stabilizes as parts of the host cell genome when inserted into host mesenchymal cells after reverse transcription. In addition to the host cell division, the viral genome also replicates during the DNA replication cycle. Tyrosine-protein kinase transforming protein Fps encoded by v-fps has the ability to induce transformation by promoting tyrosine phosphorylation of the PDGFbeta receptor [3, 4]. Thus, the Japanese scientists have greatly contributed to the field during the early days of oncology research.

1.2 Viral genome integration

Retroviral integration is a type of insertional mutagenesis. Integration processes are widely studied from biochemistry, and their molecular mechanisms are elucidated. Retrovirus-induced tumorigenesis is divided into two types. First, the retroviral genome carries the oncogene such as *v-onc*, and the inserted viral element may induce malignant tumors. Second, the inserted retroviral element has the promoter or enhancer activity of the host proto-oncogene. The genome of human papilloma virus (HPV), hepatitis B virus (HBV), human T-cell adult leukemia virus (HTLV) [5], avian sarcoma virus (ASV) [6], feline leukemia virus (FeLV) [7], murine leukemia virus (MLV) [8–13], and mouse mammary tumor virus (MMTV) can be integrated in the host genome. As a survival strategy, the inserted retroviral genome (provirus) is thereafter replicated during host cell division.

The retroviral promoter and enhancer elements in LTRs originally promote the expression of retroviral genes such as *gag*, *env*, and *pol* [14] (**Figure 1**). However, once integrated in the host genome, LTR elements can promote host gene expression in place of the host genome promoters and enhancers. After infection, the retroviral RNA genome is reverse-transcribed into DNA, which forms a pre-insertion complex (PIC) with the oligomeric integrase enzyme [15], which catalyzes the insertion reaction. The PIC crosses the nuclear envelope through the nuclear pore complex to access host cell DNA. The retroviral DNA ends then attack and nick the host DNA with target nucleotides. These ends are ligated to the truncated host DNA to complete the insertion process involving replication of the target nucleotides.

To date, extensive research has been conducted on target motifs for retroviral insertion to better understand tumorigenesis, neuronal damage, aging, and immunodeficiency including acquired immunodeficiency syndrome (AIDS). Retroviral-host DNA interactions support specific host DNA structures [16–21] but are less likely to be inserted into particular base sequences. Previous studies on human immunodeficiency virus (HIV)-1 insertion have shown that the insertion sites are distributed in 10-bp cycles on the nucleosome surface of the outward DNA major groove of chromatin [16, 22].

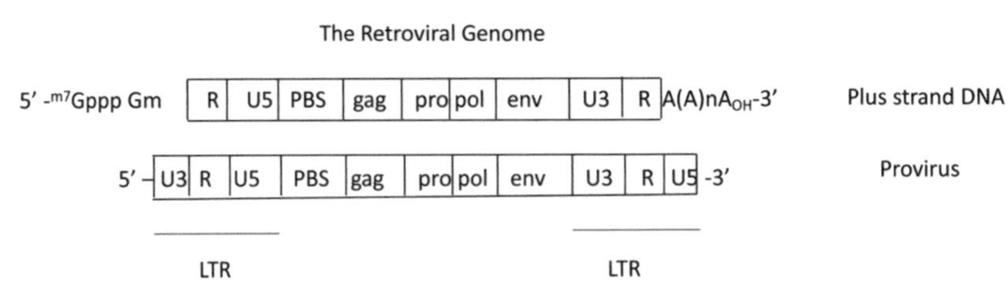

Figure 1.
A common structure of the retroviral genome. Plus strand RNA is shown. R, terminal redundant sequence; U5, unique 5′ sequence; PBS, tRNA primer-binding site; gag, group-specific antigen encoding capsid protein MA (matrix), CA, capsid protein; NC, nucleocapsid; pro, protease; pol, polymerase including reverse transcriptase (RT) and integrase (IN) catalyzing integration; env, envelope glycoproteins; U3, unique 3′ sequence. U3, R, and U5 are duplicated at both ends of the DNA provirus genome in the host genome sequence to form the long terminal repeat (LTR). LTR is essential for the initiation of viral DNA syntheses by reverse transcription as well as the integration of proviral DNA and the regulation of viral gene expression.

2. HPV

HPV is one of the most common viruses that infect more than half women once in life through sexual intercourse. It is a small DNA virus with approximately 8000 bp circular double-stranded DNA in its genome. The viral particle has icosahedral capsid structure as its outer shell. The virus has been known to be involved in the development of cervical, anal, and vaginal cancer and condyloma acuminatum. Many types of HPV are known, and high-risk HPV based on this cancer risk is concentrated in specific subgroups epidemiologically. In particular, types 16 and 18 have high carcinogenic risks of cervical intraepithelial neoplasia (CIN) and cancer. Type 16 has been detected in the Japanese 5-year-old girls [23]. High-risk group (types 16, 18, 31, 33, 35, 39, 45, 51, 52, 56, 58, 59, and 68) causes bladder cancer and pharyngeal cancer in addition to vulvar and cervical cancer. Low-risk group (HPV2, 27, and 57) causes verruca vulgaris that develops in the hands and feet [24].

HPV genome has early genes (E1, E2, E4, E5, E6, and E7) and late genes encoding viral capsid proteins (L1 and L2). E6 and E7 are considered to be involved in carcinogenesis. E6 binds to a tumor-suppressor gene product p53 and degrades p53 through promoting the ubiquitination. It also contributes to carcinogenesis by reactivating telomerase reverse transcriptase (hTERT) and degrading proteins with PDZ domain [shared by—post-synaptic density protein (PSD95), Drosophila disc large tumor suppressor (Dlg1), and Zonula occludens-1 protein (zo-1)]. E7 binds to the tumor suppressor gene pRb and contributes to carcinogenesis by releasing and activating the transcription factor E2F bound to pRb. It is also involved in carcinogenesis by interacting with cyclin-dependent kinase (Cdk) inhibitors p21 and p27 to evade cell cycle checkpoint mechanisms and apoptosis. However, in many cases, immortalization does not occur only by the actions of human cervix mucosal cells E6 and E7. In the well-known HeLa cell line, telomerase is activated, preventing the gradual shortening of telomeres in cell death.

High-risk HPV can be detected in more than 90% patients suffering from cervical cancer and dysplasia, which is a precancerous lesion, and in the vulva of 5% normal women. Although HPV is also integrated into the genome of host cells, its integration pattern has unique features. The E6 and E7 genes are retained in the provirus with frequent deletion mutations in E2 gene. Thus, the viral genome is also found to be truncated in the complex reaction of integration, but its carcinogenicity is rather enhanced. Low-grade dysplasia of the cervix and cervical intraepithelial neoplasia (CIN) is well known. These pathological changes are reversible and are known to spontaneously disappear within about 3 years. However, about 10% infected patients sustain the infection for more than 3 years, and cervical cancer occurs after several months to several decades in some of them. HPV genome is integrated into the host cell genome during the progression of CIN, and the progression becomes irreversible.

2.1 Clinical test for HPV detection

HPV-DNA typing tests have been conducted using real-time PCR, loop-mediated isothermal amplification (LAMP) [25, 26], invader, and hybridization methods. In recent years, the Clinichip method [27] combining LAMP is broadly available in advanced countries including Japan due to the ability to amplify genes at a constant temperature. The LAMP method is very specific because it uses four primers to recognize the six regions of the HPV genome. Nonspecific amplification does not occur because the amplification reaction depends on the order of the six regions of the HPV gene. In addition, since the amplification product constitutes the target gene sequence, the target gene can be detected immediately by the presence or absence of amplification.

In an environment where electricity availability is limited, easy-to-use and durable reagents and equipment are desirable. In recent years, attempts have been made to spread virus testing as point-of-care tests (POCT) [28]. For some pathogens such as malarial parasite (*Plasmodium*), HIV, Ebola virus, and Zika virus, development of the testing system by fluid device is in progress; however, HPV detection methods have not been put to practical use as POCT yet.

3. HBV

HBV has been identified as the pathogen that causes acute and chronic hepatitis B [29, 30]. HBV is a DNA hepatitis virus and has a double structure of an envelope and a core. In persistent infections, the HBV genome is often inserted into the hepatocyte genome and is not eliminated by the host's immune system. Several studies on many common insertion sites have identified common integration sites in the HBV genome by full genome sequence of hepatocellular carcinoma [31]. The envelope protein of HBV covers the HBs antigen, and the core protein is called the HBc antigen. HBV DNA encodes HBs antigen, HBc antigen, X protein, and DNA polymerase. The HBe antigen is translated from the pre-C gene and the downstream HBc antigen. It is released into blood as a soluble protein during HBV virus growth and therefore considered a marker for the virus growth. In asymptomatic carriers positive for HBe antigen, the host immune system continuously reacts with HBV-infected hepatocytes, and biopsy reports show persistent lymphocyte infiltration in the portal vascular area of liver tissues. If the damage persists for a long time, remodeling of the hepatocytes occurs and progresses to cirrhosis with obvious fibrotic crosslinks. After all, when seroconversion occurs in HBV carriers negative for HBe antigen and positive for HBe antibody, the patient becomes an inactive carrier. HBV particles remain alive during periods of inactivity. Host immune system can attack infected hepatocytes, and hepatocyte regeneration may occur with genomic mutations, and the effects of the inserted HBV genome persist. Hepatocellular carcinoma can develop with persistent liver dysfunction associated with liver cirrhosis.

3.1 Clinical test for HBV detection

For the diagnosis of hepatitis B, HBs antigen/antibody, HBc antibody, HBe antigen/antibody, and HBV DNA are detected, and HBV DNA polymerase activity is measured. HBs antigen is produced continuously in patients with HBV infection; thus, positive results for HBe antigen can diagnose current infection with HBV. Recently, the HBs antigen measurement system has become very sensitive, and infected people have been found to be positive for HBs. In addition to antigen or antibody detection method, viral DNA detection system (quantitative PCR, LAMP method) has been used for clinical tests. Liver fibrosis is seen as a precancerous stage of HBV and hepatitis C virus (HCV) infection. Liver biopsy and qualitative analysis of hyaluronic acid and type IV collagen in blood are well-known methods to evaluate liver fibrosis progress. Monitoring of glycolysis of serum M2BP (Macingo binding biomarker) is used to evaluate liver fibrotic stage [32]. Recent studies have suggested that the most common cause of nonexclusion of HBV is covalently closed circular DNA (cccDNA). When HBV infects hepatocytes, the incomplete duplex circular DNA genome becomes a complete duplex and is retained in the nucleus in the form of cccDNA. This HBV gene is the source of HBV replication. Since cccDNA is an extremely stable biochemical structure, it can be used as a monitoring marker after the infection. As the nucleic acid analog drug has little effect on reducing HBV cccDNA, a high risk of reactivation remains. If host immunity is suppressed, the reactivation occurs from this cccDNA as a starting transcriptional point. Therefore, elimination or suppression of reactivation will be central to future therapeutic strategies [33].

In the clinical tests for HBV detection, the detection sensitivity of the enzyme-linked immunosorbent assay (ELISA) method for HBs antigen is higher than those of other tests. Each available method depends on the titer of the used antibody, and the sensitivity varies. In particular, the mutation in the gene encoding the envelope protein HBs antigen may cause false negative results. Many test kits increase sensitivity by using multiple monoclonal antibodies or a polyclonal antibody that has an affinity for multiple epitopes. In some cases, antibodies that recognize epitopes within the viral particle are used instead of surface proteins with many mutations. However, the high sensitivity of many kits may instead cause false positive results. Accordingly, actual early diagnosis requires careful evaluation of test results in combination with other clinical tests.

4. HTLV type 1 (HTLV-1)

Another important human carcinogenic virus is human T-cell leukemia virus type 1 (HTLV-1). This virus has the potential to cause adult T-cell leukemia/lymphoma (ATL), HTLV-1-associated myelopathy (HAM), and HTLV-1 uveitis (HU). These diseases develop in HTLV-1 carriers after prolonged latent infection. HTLV-1 carriers are particularly prevalent in southwest Japan, including Kyushu, Shikoku, and Okinawa. HTLV-1 was isolated and reported by Gallo R as the first human pathogenic retrovirus in 1980. Yorio Hinuma of Kyoto University in Japan precisely analyzed the genomic structure and identified the HTLV-1 [34]. HTLV-1 is a weakly infective virus particle, and cell-to-cell transmission is the main route of infection.

4.1 Molecular biology of HTLV-1

ATL is a hematologic malignancy in which abnormal lymphocytes appear in peripheral blood and infiltrate various organs throughout the body. Kiyoshi Takatsuki of Kumamoto University in Japan and Taku Uchiyama of Kyoto University collected samples. In 1981, Hinuma identified HTLV-1 to be the causative virus of ATL; this was the first report on tumor-induced retrovirus in humans. Most infected cells are CD4 + CD25 + T cells. Viral receptors are thought to involve other proteins and heparan sulfate. HTLV-1 is an approximately spherical virus particle about 100 nm in diameter and has an envelope. It has an RNA genome composed of the genes common to retroviruses such as *gag*, *pro*, *pol*, and *env*, as well as the gene encoding pX. It selectively uses the splicing and translation initiation sites in a region less than 2 kb called pX located between the env gene and the 3′ LTR [35] and uses the plus and minus strands relative to the transcription direction and efficiently. It often encodes several regulatory and accessory genes. As described later, this pX is involved in the action of HTLV-1 encoding HTLV-1 bZIP factor (HBZ).

Tax and HBZ may be the carcinogenic potentials of HTLV-1. Tax is a potent transactivator essential for the activation of the viral promoter 5′ LTR. After entering the cell by infection, the virus particle capsid is lost, and the HTLV-1 genomic RNA is reverse transcribed to form genomic duplex DNA. Thereafter, the integrase encoded by the viral genome and the DNA end forms a complex, which contacts the genomic DNA on the cell side, and inserts by catalytic reaction. The 5-base-long sequence of the targeted host cell genome is duplicated at both ends of the inserted viral genome in the insertion process. Tax, the transcript of TLV-1 regulatory gene tax, not only binds to the HTLV-1 promoter to promote viral transcription and expression but also interacts with cell-side transcription factors to activate host gene transcription activity. Therefore, *tax* is implicated in the early stages of tumorigenesis of infected cells. However, in peripheral blood of most ATL patients, Tax is suppressed by its promoter 5′ LTR deletion and epigenetic modification. Thus, Tax is not essential, at least at the final stage of carcinogenesis. Recently, Matsuoka has suggested that Tax is constitutively expressed in a small fraction of leukemia cells, and this fraction triggers an anti-apoptotic mechanism to establish sustained infection and induces oncogenesis [36]. Tax is induced by a variety of cytotoxic stresses and also promotes HTLV-1 replication. Thus, it protects infected cells from apoptosis and increases the chance of viral infection at the critical phase of disease in the carrier. Another HBZ gene is expressed in all ATL patients causing and promoting the growth of ATL cells; therefore, it may be the gene responsible for ATL.

4.2 Insertion site of HTLV-1

At present, in addition to the carcinogenesis by the proteins of these viruses themselves, attention has been focused on the activation of host genes at the insertion site. The integrated HTLV-1 provirus has the LTR [35] in both directions for the transcription. This sequence has many motifs that bind to transcription factors on the host and have strong promoter/enhancer activities. Therefore, there may be an increase in constitutive expression of the gene at the insertion site. Ogawa performed systematic genome analysis of ATL cells in 426 ATL patients and showed that genes interacting with Tax, T-cell receptor-NF-κB signal transduction, T-cell transport, and other T-cell-related pathways as well as genes related to immune surveillance are injured by the integration. Also, the expressions of VAV1, IRF4, and FYN related to lymphocyte maturation and signal transduction, chemokine receptors CCR4 and CCR7, and gene fusions (CTLA4-CD28 and ICOS-CD28) were enhanced in the infected cells [37]. Viral transcripts were mainly derived from the antisense strand. Also, the suppression of *Tax* expression and the constitutive expression of *HBZ* were observed in almost all patients. These insertion sites have not been known to be likely to occur in any particular sequence motif.

4.3 Clinical test for HTLV-1 detection

To date, no chromosomal abnormality specific to HTLV-1 has been observed, and Southern blot or inverse PCR methods are used for diagnosis; however, in recent years, multiplex LAMP (RT-LAMP) using universal probe has been developed. The method detects both HIV and HTLV-1 RNA from the same sample [39]. HAS HTLV-1 analyzing system (HAS)-Flow method has also been proposed to evaluate the progression of ATL stage by applying flow cytometric analysis focusing on surface markers of infected immune cells [38].

5. Integration model in mice lymphomas

5.1 The specificity of insertion sequence of the retrovirus genome

As experimental models of MLV integration, BXH2 [40], AKXD [41–44], and SL/Kh [20, 45–52] are well-known mouse strains into which endogenous provirus genomes have been inserted. The genome of an endogenous MLV, AKV [14], was integrated into *gltscr 1* [20], which has been characterized as a tumor suppressor gene. This locus was identified as *emv11* on chr 7. In our previous work, the inserted AKV genome was shown to contain the full-length MLV genome and expressed to form a retroviral particle, which had the ability to infect lymphocytes according to its retroviral tropism. In the consequent tumorigenesis, the phenotype of the murine tumor is generally variable in inbred strains. For example, AKR/J mice are susceptible to T-cell lymphoma/leukemia [53–55]; however, in BXH2 mice [39, 40], tumors resemble myeloid and lymphocytic tumors. Even if the MLV is integrated into identical genes, the tumor phenotypes are variable [56]. It is likely that the individual genetic backgrounds of the inbred mouse strains determine the phenotype in combination with the integration-induced expression of oncogenes. Thus, oncogenes are responsible for the tumorigenesis; however, the phenotypes of the tumors are determined by other elements, including the genetic background. The insertion site of MLV has been studied using model mouse strains. SL/Kh strain is known to be a model of acute lymphocytic leukemia/lymphoma by MLV infection, and the target sequence of integration has been identified. This phenomenon may not always be generalized in human retroviruses as MLV LTR is very long and has palindromic motifs unlike HTLV-1 LTR. This sequence motif may contribute to the stabilization of the structure as the tetrameric integrase binds to the LTR. Such a stabilizing structure is not found in HTLV-1, and the retroviral genome may differ in HTLV-1 and MLV in this regard. The existence of a specific sequence motif in the genome insertion of the virus has been the subject of much debate and was initially resolved negatively in early days. The conclusion was that a virus integration is a random event [57] (by Howard Temin, who discovered reverse transcriptase and won the Nobel Prize in 1975). The randomness was proved through the genome analysis of infecting fibroblasts with integrated MLV in the culture state artificially. No common sequence motif for the insertion site was found in this way. However, there has been a report that active transcriptional genes can be the target of integration [21]. Besides, there are reports stating that palindrome sequence is favored by integration [16, 58]; however, the target sequence itself is yet to be identified. The idea is that viral insertion affects the transcriptional activity of the host cell genome by the three-dimensional structure of chromatin. A model may be considered in which the integrase complex binds to the site where DNA is locally released during transcription.

To study MLV genome insertion *in vivo,* inbred strains of mice harboring many copies of endogenous MLV genomes were developed. SL/Kh is one of the inbred strains (Tsukuba, Japan; http://www.riken.jp/engn/index.html) [14, 45]. In this strain, the harbored MLV genome is spontaneously and selectively integrated into the genome of the B-cell genome DNA. In reference to the data about MLV insertion sites in the genome of SL/Kh mice, whether MLV insertion occurred preferentially into the specific sequence motifs in the host cell genome was investigated. *Stat5a* [20, 51, 59, 60] and *c-myc* [47] were the target genes for MLV insertion. More than 95% studied SL/Kh mice had such the MLV genome (AKV) insertion in zinc finger protein 521 gene (*Zfp521*) in the genomic DNA of B-cell lineage at 7 weeks of age [61] (**Figure 2**).

5.2 Integration target sequence

To date, such significantly selective insertion into the specific gene has not been known. When insertion further occurs in an oncogene (e.g., *Stat5a* [51] or *c-myc* [47]) in addition to *Zfp521* in the genome of SL/Kh mice, B lymphocytic leukemia develops.

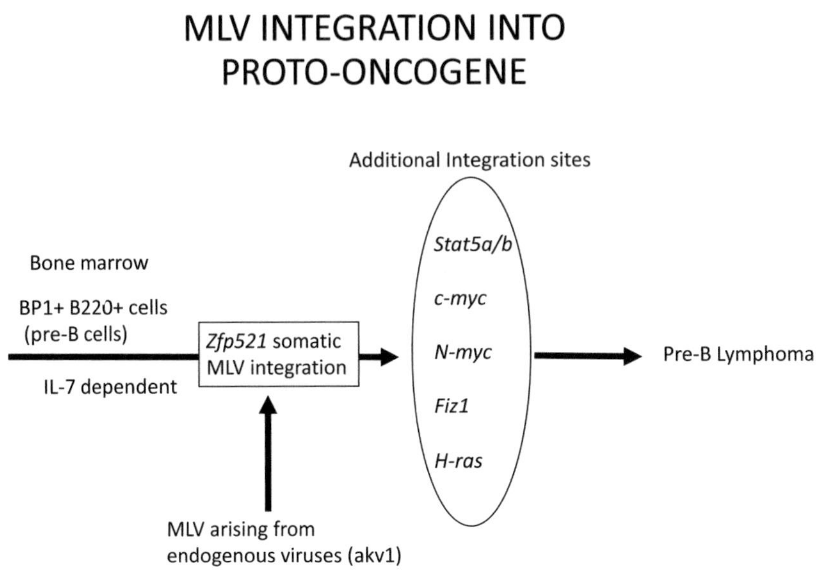

Figure 2.
Murine leukemia retrovirus (MLV) integration into oncogenes in SL/Kh lymphoma. In most cases of lymphoma, MLV integrations into more than one oncogenes, including Stat5a, c-myc, Fiz1, Hipk2, and others, are observed. It is not clear why the tumor cells are restricted to pre-B lymphoma phenotype. To date, genetic background dependent on Bomb1 is critical for conferring the phenotype. In addition, Stat5a and Zfp521 genes cooperate with IL-7 and pre-B cell receptor signal pathways, respectively. Host cell phenotype at the integration may contribute to the phenotypes. Differentiation stage of the host cell at the mutagenesis may be one of the critical factors of the phenotype.

In AKXD and SL/Kh lymphoma genome, *Zfp521* is one of the most frequent targets of MLV integration [62]. This gene locus was first reported as a common integration site, ecotropic retrovirus integration site 3 (*Evi3*) [61–64]. In more than 400 male SL/Kh mice, >90% pre-B-lymphoma genomes acquired the integrated proviral genome within a 50-bp segment located in the region of the second to third exon of *Zfp521*. This target gene carries alternating palindrome sequences [16], which was frequently targeted by MLV insertion. *Zfp521* is one the novel identified target genes. It probably contributes to chondrocyte development [65], in addition to B-cell development that requires an abnormal chimeric gene [64]. Each insertion occurs once or twice during the development of lymphoma within a 50-bp segment located in the second intron to the third exon of *Zfp521*. Most commonly, the insertion occurs at the ":" site in the sequence "CTGAATTG*AAAC:* AACTTCAGC*TGTTT*," where the pair of underlined sequences and the pair of sequences in italics are palindromic sequences [61–63, 66]. The insertion does not occur randomly; they frequently occur at approximately 10-bp intervals and are symmetrically distributed within the shown 50-bp segment (**Figure 3**).

SL/Kh mouse has multiple copies of the endogenous virus, which produces viral particles and infects immature B-cell lineages suitable for tropism. Several common insertion sites such as Stat5a and Stat5b and well-known genes such as c-myc have been identified till date. Interestingly, many of these insertions occur upstream of the translational initiation site of the protein, so that many intact targeted proteins are produced. The fact that many insertions occur in such specific genes suggests that DNA structures such as palindromic sequences are targeted. However, insertions in a short 50-bp segment cannot have such secondary structure. MLV insertion was observed in almost the entire genome of this SL/Kh acute lymphocytic leukemia/lymphoma. The integration target segment is located just before the translation initiation

DOI: http://dx.doi.org/10.5772/intechopen.89331

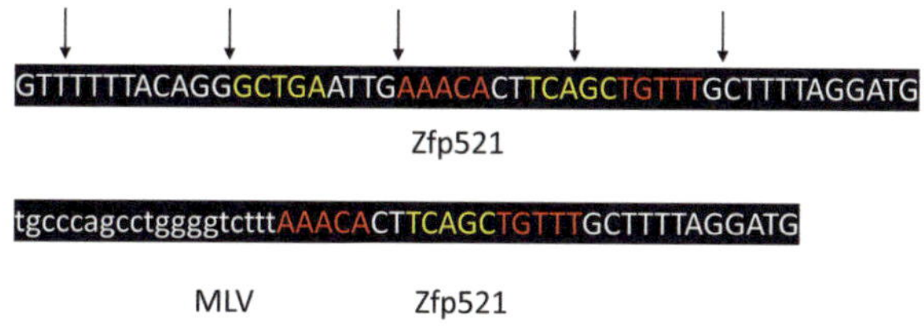

Figure 3.
Alternate palindrome sequence in Zfp521. The upper and lower sequences represent the native sequence of host murine Zfp521 gene and the junction sequence of host murine Zfp521 gene with the integrated MLV genome, respectively. Green and red letters represent pairs of alternating palindromes. The sequences in the same colors are palindromes. The downward arrows represent the hot spot of the MLV integration.

origin of the Zfp521 gene, which was first reported as a retrovirus insertion sequence. As a result of the insertion, downstream Zfp521 gene is constitutively expressed, and the upregulation may be responsible for acute lymphocytic leukemia/lymphoma.

5.3 Interaction partners for MLV integrase and recent developments in the biosafety of gene therapy

Recently, several cellular proteins including transcription regulatory factors and chromatin and RNA-binding proteins have been discovered as potential interaction partners for MLV integrase [67]. The bromodomain and extra-terminal domain (BET)-containing family of proteins (BRD2, BRD3, BRD4, and BRDT) act as cellular-binding partners of MLV integrase and preferentially bind to open chromatin regions that are enriched for transcription start sites, CpG islands, DNase I-hypersensitive sites, and proto-oncogenes [68–73]. The BET family of proteins plays a critical role in regulating gene transcription through epigenetic interactions between dual bromodomains and acetylated lysines on histones H3 and H4 during cellular proliferation, cell cycle progression, and differentiation processes [8, 9]. *In vitro* interaction analysis in human cells revealed that the ET domain of BRDs, BRD4 in particular, interacts with a motif in the unstructured C-terminal tail of MLV integrase, and these interactions are crucial for the recruitment of the MLV PIC to host DNA during integration [10, 11]. Through the recognition of open chromatin structure, BET proteins have been suggested to contribute to the tethering of the MLV PIC to the host chromatin [10, 12]. Furthermore, it has been shown that the cell-permeable small molecule JQ-1, a pan-BET bromodomain inhibitor, prevents the BRD4-acetylated lysine interaction by competitively binding to BRD4 and reduces MLV integration frequencies at transcription start sites [4, 13, 14]. These findings suggest that BET proteins navigate the MLV genome and promote efficient MLV integration around transcription start sites associated with a chromatin structure characteristic of an open, transcriptionally active domain [3].

The dual bromodomain protein of BRD2 promotes B-cell expansion and plays a critical role in the regulation of mitogenic response genes, particularly cyclin A, in B cells [15]. In addition, it has been shown that the inhibition of BRD4 leads to the suppression of germinal center B-cell differentiation and antibody responses through the down-regulation of nuclear factor-κBp65 activation and B-cell lymphoma 6 expression [16]. Hence, these BET proteins might broadly contribute to tumorigenesis in cooperation with MLV integration in spontaneous B-cell lymphoma development, and these findings likely provide novel standpoints of proto-oncogene function as well as a better understanding of MLV insertional mutagenesis [15, 17].

The stable integration of retroviral vectors is suitable to deliver therapeutic genes into cells to correct genetic diseases. MLV-based retroviral vectors are one of the most frequently used gene delivery vehicles in gene therapy studies for primary immunodeficiencies such as adenosine deaminase deficiency-severe combined immunodeficiency [10, 18, 19]. However, a subset of patients developed serious adverse events including leukemia that could be attributed to the integration pattern and vector design [10, 18]. MLV-based retroviral vectors integrate in the vicinity of transcription start site through the interaction between the C-terminal tail of MLV integrase (amino acids 381–408) and the ET domain of BET family of proteins [18, 20]. To resolve side effects such as leukemia, BET-independent MLV vectors have been developed by truncation of the C-terminal tail of MLV integrase or the single W390A mutation [18, 20]. Most recently, next-generation BET-independent MLV vectors have been engineered with the addition of the chromodomain of Chromobox protein homolog 1 (CBX1) to MLV integrase$_{\text{_W390A}}$. The MLV integrase$_{\text{_W390A-CBX1}}$ efficiently targets integration away from traditional markers of MLV integration including gene regulatory elements [10]. These findings open new avenues to improve the biosafety of gammaretroviral vectors for gene therapy.

6. Summary

We followed the history of viral carcinogenic research in this review. The topic of viral carcinogenesis mentioned here is a case where the viral genome is inserted into the host genome. Because the molecular mechanism of viral carcinogenesis has been elucidated, significant novel technical methods will be developed in the future.

Clinical sequence analyzes gene changes occurring at diseased sites and provides information useful for diagnosis and treatment of diseases based on the results of gene mutations.

In addition to the various nucleic acid analysis methods such as conventional PCR and LAMP, next-generation sequencing and other rapid technological innovation will aid in the measurement and analysis of numerous gene sequences in a short period. Furthermore, these technologies are expected to be used in the future to analyze infectious diseases such as cancer virus types, HPV high-risk groups, and virus insertion sites. Information on cancer virus infection will also be valuable for designing personalized drugs for cancer patients in the future.

Acknowledgements

This work was supported by a Grant-in-Aid from the Ministry of Education, Culture, Sports, Science, and Technology of Japan (no. 15H05721) and a Grant-in-Aid from the Scientific Research on Innovative Areas, MEXT, Japan (no. P2013-201).

Conflicts of interest

The authors declare no conflicts of interest.

Abbreviations

HPV	human papilloma virus
HBV	hepatitis B virus
HTLV-1	human T-cell leukemia virus type 1
MLV	murine leukemia virus

Author details

Tatsuaki Tsuruyama*, Shuichiro Ogawa and Norishige Yamada
Department of Drug and Discovery Medicine, Clinical Bioresource Center of Kyoto University Hospital, Sakyo-ku, Kyoto, Japan

*Address all correspondence to: tsuruyam@kuhp.kyoto-u.ac.jp

References

[1] Hanafusa T, Wang LH, Anderson SM, Karess RE, Hayward WS, Hanafusa H. Characterization of the transforming gene of Fujinami sarcoma virus. Proceedings of the National Academy of Sciences of the United States of America. 1980;**77**(5):3009-3013. DOI: 10.1073/pnas.77.5.3009

[2] Mathey-Prevot B, Shibuya M, Samarut J, Hanafusa H. Revertants and partial transformants of rat fibroblasts infected with Fujinami sarcoma virus. Journal of Virology. 1984;**50**(2):325-334

[3] Anderson DH, Ismail PM. v-fps causes transformation by inducing tyrosine phosphorylation and activation of the PDGFbeta receptor. Oncogene. 1998;**16**(18):2321-2331. DOI: 10.1038/sj.onc.1201780

[4] Wang Y, Li J, Li Y, Fang L, Sun X, Chang S, et al. Identification of ALV-J associated acutely transforming virus Fu-J carrying complete v-fps oncogene. Virus Genes. 2016;**52**(3):365-371. DOI: 10.1007/s11262-016-1301-6

[5] Derse D, Crise B, Li Y, Princler G, Lum N, Stewart C, et al. Human T-cell leukemia virus type 1 integration target sites in the human genome: Comparison with those of other retroviruses. Journal of Virology. 2007;**81**(12):6731-6741. DOI: 10.1128/Jvi.02752-06

[6] Aiyar A, Hindmarsh P, Skalka AM, Leis J. Concerted integration of linear retroviral DNA by the avian sarcoma virus integrase in vitro: Dependence on both long terminal repeat termini. Journal of Virology. 1996;**70**(6):3571-3580

[7] Levy LS, Lobelle-Rich PA, Overbaugh J. flvi-2, a target of retroviral insertional mutagenesis in feline thymic lymphosarcomas, encodes bmi-1. Oncogene. 1993;**8**(7):1833-1838

[8] Beverly LJ, Capobianco AJ. Perturbation of Ikaros isoform selection by MLV integration is a cooperative event in Notch(IC)-induced T cell leukemogenesis. Cancer Cell. 2003;**3**(6):551-564

[9] Hematti P, Hong BK, Ferguson C, Adler R, Hanawa H, Sellers S, et al. Distinct genomic integration of MLV and SIV vectors in primate hematopoietic stem and progenitor cells. PLoS Biology. 2004;**2**(12):e423. DOI: 10.1371/journal.pbio.0020423

[10] Jeanteur P. Differences in the MLV and HIV-1 integration sites could be important for gene therapy. Bulletin du Cancer. 2003;**90**(8-9):671

[11] LaFave MC, Varshney GK, Gildea DE, Wolfsberg TG, Baxevanis AD, Burgess SM. MLV integration site selection is driven by strong enhancers and active promoters. Nucleic Acids Research. 2014;**42**(7):4257-4269. DOI: 10.1093/nar/gkt1399

[12] Schambach A. Toward a safer integration profile of MLV-based retroviral vectors. Molecular Therapy. 2014;**22**(8):1405-1406. DOI: 10.1038/mt.2014.124

[13] Tsuruyama T, Hiratsuka T, Yamada N. Hotspots of MLV integration in the hematopoietic tumor genome. Oncogene. 2017;**36**(9):1169-1175. DOI: 10.1038/onc.2016.285

[14] Lenz J, Crowther R, Straceski A, Haseltine W. Nucleotide sequence of the Akv env gene. Journal of Virology. 1982;**42**(2):519-529

[15] Elis E, Ehrlich M, Prizan-Ravid A, Laham-Karam N, Bacharach E. p12 tethers the murine leukemia virus pre-integration complex to mitotic

chromosomes. PLoS Pathogens. 2012;**8**(12):e1003103. DOI: 10.1371/journal.ppat.1003103

[16] Holman AG, Coffin JM. Symmetrical base preferences surrounding HIV-1, avian sarcoma/leukosis virus, and murine leukemia virus integration sites. Proceedings of the National Academy of Sciences of the United States of America. 2005;**102**(17):6103-6107. DOI: 10.1073/pnas.0501646102

[17] Lewinski MK, Yamashita M, Emerman M, Ciuffi A, Marshall H, Crawford G, et al. Retroviral DNA integration: Viral and cellular determinants of target-site selection. PLOS Pathogens. 2006;**2**(6):e60. DOI: 10.1371/journal.ppat.0020060

[18] Pruss D, Reeves R, Bushman FD, Wolffe AP. The influence of DNA and nucleosome structure on integration events directed by HIV integrase. The Journal of Biological Chemistry. 1994;**269**(40):25031-25041

[19] Schröder AR, Shinn P, Chen H, Berry C, Ecker JR, Bushman F. HIV-1 integration in the human genome favors active genes and local hotspots. Cell. 2002;**110**(4):521-529. DOI: 10.1016/s0092-8674(02)00864-4

[20] Tsuruyama T, Hiratsuka T, Jin G, Imai Y, Takeuchi H, Maruyama Y, et al. Murine leukemia retrovirus integration induces the formation of transcription factor complexes on palindromic sequences in the signal transducer and activator of transcription factor 5a gene during the development of pre-B lymphomagenesis. American Journal of Pathology. 2011;**178**(3):1374-1386. DOI: 10.1016/j.ajpath.2010.12.012

[21] Wu XL, Li Y, Crise B, Burgess SM. Transcription start regions in the human genome are favored targets for MLV integration. Science. 2003;**300**(5626):1749-1751

[22] Wang GP, Ciuffi A, Leipzig J, Berry CC, Bushman FD. HIV integration site selection: Analysis by massively parallel pyrosequencing reveals association with epigenetic modifications. Genome Research. 2007;**17**(8):1186-1194. DOI: 10.1101/gr.6286907

[23] Kojima A, Maeda H, Kurahashi N, Sakagami G, Kubo K, Yoshimoto H, et al. Human papillomaviruses in the normal oral cavity of children in Japan. Oral Oncology. 2003;**39**(8):821-828

[24] de Martel C, Ferlay J, Franceschi S, Vignat J, Bray F, Forman D, et al. Global burden of cancers attributable to infections in 2008: A review and synthetic analysis. The Lancet Oncology. 2012;**13**(6):607-615. DOI: 10.1016/S1470-2045(12)70137-7

[25] Nagamine K, Kuzuhara Y, Notomi T. Isolation of single-stranded DNA from loop-mediated isothermal amplification products. Biochemical and Biophysical Research Communications. 2002;**290**(4):1195-1198. DOI: 10.1006/bbrc.2001.6334

[26] Notomi T, Okayama H, Masubuchi H, Yonekawa T, Watanabe K, Amino N, et al. Loop-mediated isothermal amplification of DNA. Nucleic Acids Research. 2000;**28**(12):E63. DOI: 10.1093/nar/28.12.e63

[27] Satoh T, Matsumoto K, Fujii T, Sato O, Gemma N, Onuki M, et al. Rapid genotyping of carcinogenic human papillomavirus by loop-mediated isothermal amplification using a new automated DNA test (Clinichip HPV™). Journal of Virological Methods. 2013;**188**(1-2):83-93. DOI: 10.1016/j.jviromet.2012.10.014

[28] Chen H, Liu K, Li Z, Wang P. Point of care testing for infectious diseases. Clinica Chimica Acta. 2019;**493**:138-147. DOI: 10.1016/j.cca.2019.03.008

[29] Purcell RH, Gerin JL, Almeida JB, Holland PV. Radioimmunoassay for the detection of the core of the Dane particle and antibody to it. Intervirology. 1974;**2**(4):231-243. DOI: 10.1159/000149428

[30] Zavalin A, Todd EM, Rawhouser PD, Yang J, Norris JL, Caprioli RM. Direct imaging of single cells and tissue at sub-cellular spatial resolution using transmission geometry MALDI MS. Journal of Mass Spectrometry. 2012;**47**(11):i. DOI: 10.1002/jms.3132

[31] Furuta M, Tanaka H, Shiraishi Y, Unida T, Imamura M, Fujimoto A, et al. Characterization of HBV integration patterns and timing in liver cancer and HBV-infected livers. Oncotarget. 2018;**9**(38):25075-25088. DOI: 10.18632/oncotarget.25308

[32] Kuno A, Ikehara Y, Tanaka Y, Ito K, Matsuda A, Sekiya S, et al. A serum "sweet-doughnut" protein facilitates fibrosis evaluation and therapy assessment in patients with viral hepatitis. Scientific Reports. 2013;**3**:1065. DOI: 10.1038/srep01065

[33] Gane EJ. Future anti-HBV strategies. Liver International. 2017;**37**(Suppl 1):40-44. DOI: 10.1111/liv.13304

[34] Ishida T, Hinuma Y. The origin of Japanese HTLV-I. Nature. 1986;**322**(6079):504. DOI: 10.1038/322504a0

[35] Ruiz-Herguido C, Guiu J, D'Altri T, Inglés-Esteve J, Dzierzak E, Espinosa L, et al. Hematopoietic stem cell development requires transient Wnt/beta-catenin activity. The Journal of Experimental Medicine. 2012;**209**(8):1457-1468. DOI: 10.1084/jem.20120225

[36] Caginalp C, Caginalp G. Opinion: Valuation, liquidity price, and stability of cryptocurrencies. Proceedings of the National Academy of Sciences of the United States of America. 2018;**115**(6):1131-1134. DOI: 10.1073/pnas.1722031115

[37] Kataoka K, Nagata Y, Kitanaka A, Shiraishi Y, Shimamura T, Yasunaga J, et al. Integrated molecular analysis of adult T cell leukemia/lymphoma. Nature Genetics. 2015;**47**(11):1304-1315. DOI: 10.1038/ng.3415

[38] Becherer L, Bakheit M, Frischmann S, Stinco S, Borst N, Zengerle R, et al. Simplified real-time multiplex detection of loop-mediated isothermal amplification using novel mediator displacement probes with universal reporters. Analytical Chemistry. 2018;**90**(7):4741-4748. DOI: 10.1021/acs.analchem.7b05371

[39] Kobayashi S, Tian Y, Ohno N, Yuji K, Ishigaki T, Isobe M, et al. The CD3 versus CD7 plot in multicolor flow cytometry reflects progression of disease stage in patients infected with HTLV-I. PLoS One. 2013;**8**(1):e53728

[40] Shaughnessy JD Jr, Largaespada DA, Tian E, Fletcher CF, Cho BC, Vyas P, et al. Mrvi1, a common MRV integration site in BXH2 myeloid leukemias, encodes a protein with homology to a lymphoid-restricted membrane protein Jaw1. Oncogene. 1999;**18**(12):2069-2084. DOI: 10.1038/sj.onc.1202419

[41] Justice MJ, Morse HC 3rd, Jenkins NA, Copeland NG. Identification of Evi-3, a novel common site of retroviral integration in mouse AKXD B-cell lymphomas. Journal of Virology. 1994;**68**(3):1293-1300

[42] Liao X, Buchberg AM, Jenkins NA, Copeland NG. Evi-5, a common site of retroviral integration in AKXD T-cell lymphomas, maps near Gfi-1 on mouse chromosome 5. Journal of Virology. 1995;**69**(11):7132-7137

[43] Mucenski ML, Taylor BA, Ihle JN, Hartley JW, Morse HC 3rd, Jenkins NA, et al. Identification of a common ecotropic viral integration site, Evi-1, in the DNA of AKXD murine myeloid tumors. Molecular and Cellular Biology. 1988;**8**(1):301-308

[44] Mucenski ML, Taylor BA, Jenkins NA, Copeland NG. AKXD recombinant inbred strains: Models for studying the molecular genetic basis of murine lymphomas. Molecular and Cellular Biology. 1986;**6**(12):4236-4243

[45] Hiai H, Tsuruyama T, Yamada Y. Pre-B lymphomas in SL/Kh mice: A multifactorial disease model. Cancer Science. 2003;**94**(10):847-850

[46] Hiratsuka T, Tsuruyama T, Kaszynski R, Kometani K, Minato N, Nakamura T, et al. Bone marrow pre-B expansion by SL/Kh-Bomb1 locus: Not sufficient for lymphomagenesis. Leukemia Research. 2008;**32**(2):309-314. DOI: 10.1016/j.leukres.2007.05.013

[47] Jin G, Tsuruyama T, Yamada Y, Hiai H. Svi3: A provirus common integration site in c-myc in SL/Kh pre-B lymphomas. Cancer Science. 2003;**94**(9):791-795

[48] Lu LM, Shimada R, Higashi S, Zeng Z, Hiai H. Bone marrow pre-B-1 (Bomb1): A quantitative trait locus inducing bone marrow pre-B-cell expansion in lymphoma-prone SL/Kh mice. Cancer Research. 1999;**59**(11):2593-2595

[49] Okamoto K, Yamada Y, Ogawa MS, Toyokuni S, Nakakuki Y, Ikeda H, et al. Abnormal bone marrow B-cell differentiation in pre-B lymphoma-prone SL/Kh mice. Cancer Research. 1994;**54**(2):399-402

[50] Shimada MO, Yamada Y, Nakakuki Y, Okamoto K, Fukumoto M, Honjo T, et al. SL/KH strain of mice: A model of spontaneous pre-B-lymphomas. Leukemia Research. 1993;**17**(7):573-578

[51] Tsuruyama T, Nakamura T, Jin G, Ozeki M, Yamada Y, Hiai H. Constitutive activation of Stat5a by retrovirus integration in early pre-B lymphomas of SL/Kh strain mice. Proceedings of the National Academy of Sciences of the United States of America. 2002;**99**(12):8253-8258. DOI: 10.1073/pnas.112202899

[52] Yamada Y, Matsushiro H, Ogawa MS, Okamoto K, Nakakuki Y, Toyokuni S, et al. Genetic predisposition to pre-B lymphomas in SL/Kh strain mice. Cancer Research. 1994;**54**(2):403-407

[53] Haran-Ghera N, Peled A, Wu L, Shortman K, Brightman BK, Fan H. The effects of passive antiviral immunotherapy in AKR mice: I. The susceptibility of AKR mice to spontaneous and induced T cell lymphomagenesis. Leukemia. 1995;**9**(7):1199-1206

[54] Ikeda H, Rowe WP, Boyse EA, Stockert E, Sato H, Jacobs S. Relationship of infectious murine leukemia virus and virus-related antigens in genetic crosses between AKR and the Fv-1 compatible strain C57L. The Journal of Experimental Medicine. 1976;**143**(1):32-46

[55] Lenz J, Crowther R, Klimenko S, Haseltine W. Molecular cloning of a highly leukemogenic, ecotropic retrovirus from an AKR mouse. Journal of Virology. 1982;**43**(3):943-951

[56] Akagi K, Suzuki T, Stephens RM, Jenkins NA, Copeland NG. RTCGD: Retroviral tagged cancer gene database. Nucleic Acids Research. 2004;**32**(Database issue):D523-D527. DOI: 10.1093/nar/gkh013

[57] Fitts R, Temin HM. Cellular DNA surrounding integration sites of an avian retrovirus. The Journal of General Virology. 1983;**64**(2):267-274. DOI: 10.1099/0022-1317-64-2-267

[58] Coffin JM. Retroviral DNA integration. Developments in Biological Standardization. 1992;**76**:141-151

[59] Tsuruyama T, Hiratsuka T, Aini W, Nakamura T. STAT5A modulates chemokine receptor CCR6 expression and enhances pre-B cell growth in a CCL20-dependent manner. Journal of Cellular Biochemistry. 2016;**117**(11):2630-2642. DOI: 10.1002/jcb.25558

[60] Tsuruyama T, Imai Y, Takeuchi H, Hiratsuka T, Maruyama Y, Kanaya K, et al. Dual retrovirus integration tagging: Identification of new signaling molecules Fiz1 and Hipk2 that are involved in the IL-7 signaling pathway in B lymphoblastic lymphomas. Journal of Leukocyte Biology. 2010;**88**(1):107-116. DOI: 10.1189/jlb.1109748

[61] Hiratsuka T, Takei Y, Ohmori R, Imai Y, Ozeki M, Tamaki K, et al. ZFP521 contributes to pre-B-cell lymphomagenesis through modulation of the pre-B-cell receptor signaling pathway. Oncogene. 2016;**35**(25):3227-3238. DOI: 10.1038/onc.2015.385

[62] Warming S, Liu P, Suzuki T, Akagi K, Lindtner S, Pavlakis GN, et al. Evi3, a common retroviral integration site in murine B-cell lymphoma, encodes an EBFAZ-related Kruppel-like zinc finger protein. Blood. 2003;**101**(5):1934-1940. DOI: 10.1182/blood-2002-08-2652

[63] Hentges KE, Weiser KC, Schountz T, Woodward LS, Morse HC, Justice MJ. Evi3, a zinc-finger protein related to EBFAZ, regulates EBF activity in B-cell leukemia. Oncogene. 2005;**24**(7):1220-1230. DOI: 10.1038/sj.onc.1208243

[64] Yamasaki N, Miyazaki K, Nagamachi A, Koller R, Oda H, Miyazaki M, et al. Identification of Zfp521/ZNF521 as a cooperative gene for E2A-HLF to develop acute B-lineage leukemia. Oncogene. 2010;**29**(13):1963-1975. DOI: 10.1038/onc.2009.475

[65] Correa D, Hesse E, Seriwatanachai D, Kiviranta R, Saito H, Yamana K, et al. Zfp521 is a target gene and key effector of parathyroid hormone-related peptide signaling in growth plate chondrocytes. Developmental Cell. 2010;**19**(4):533-546. DOI: 10.1016/j.devcel.2010.09.008

[66] Bond HM, Mesuraca M, Carbone E, Bonelli P, Agosti V, Amodio N, et al. Early hematopoietic zinc finger protein (EHZF), the human homolog to mouse Evi3, is highly expressed in primitive human hematopoietic cells. Blood. 2004;**103**(6):2062-2070. DOI: 10.1182/blood-2003-07-2388

[67] Studamire B, Goff SP. Host proteins interacting with the Moloney murine leukemia virus integrase: Multiple transcriptional regulators and chromatin binding factors. Retrovirology. 2008;**5**:48. DOI: 10.1186/1742-4690-5-48

[68] Kvaratskhelia M, Sharma A, Larue RC, Serrao E, Engelman A. Molecular mechanisms of retroviral integration site selection. Nucleic Acids Research. 2014;**42**(16):10209-10225. DOI: 10.1093/nar/gku769

[69] Sharma A, Larue RC, Plumb MR, Malani N, Male F, Slaughter A, et al. BET proteins promote efficient murine leukemia virus integration at transcription start sites. Proceedings of the National Academy of Sciences of the United States of America. 2013;**110**(29):12036-12041. DOI: 10.1073/pnas.1307157110

[70] Dey A, Chitsaz F, Abbasi A, Misteli T, Ozato K. The double

bromodomain protein Brd4 binds to acetylated chromatin during interphase and mitosis. Proceedings of the National Academy of Sciences of the United States of America. 2003;**100**(15):8758-8763. DOI: 10.1073/pnas.1433065100

[71] Vollmuth F, Blankenfeldt W, Geyer M. Structures of the dual bromodomains of the P-TEFb-activating protein Brd4 at atomic resolution. The Journal of Biological Chemistry. 2009;**284**(52):36547-36556. DOI: 10.1074/jbc.M109.033712

[72] Umehara T, Nakamura Y, Jang MK, Nakano K, Tanaka A, Ozato K, et al. Structural basis for acetylated histone H4 recognition by the human BRD2 bromodomain. The Journal of Biological Chemistry. 2010;**285**(10):7610-7618. DOI: 10.1074/jbc.M109.062422

[73] Zhang W, Prakash C, Sum C, Gong Y, Li Y, Kwok JJ, et al. Bromodomain-containing protein 4 (BRD4) regulates RNA polymerase II serine 2 phosphorylation in human CD4+ T cells. The Journal of Biological Chemistry. 2012;**287**(51):43137-43155. DOI: 10.1074/jbc.M112.413047

Section 2

Avian Influenza - Endemic to Pandemic

Chapter 4

Prologue: Avian Influenza - An Overview from Endemic to Pandemic

Muhammad Abubakar, Abdullah Iqbal, Shumaila Manzoor and Kashif Saleemi

1. Introduction

Avian influenza also called as bird flu is an acute, contagious disease caused by Influenza A virus. Birds of order *Anseriformes* and *Charadriiformes are reservoir hosts of* influenza A viruses [1]. These viruses have the ability to infect many mammal species such as horses, pigs, cats, dogs, and humans. Influenza A viruses are negative-sense single-stranded RNA viruses with enveloped structure [2]. Influenza A viruses have shown high antigenic variability due to antigenic drift and shift phenomena. These mutation methods result in the emergence of new variants. These new variants can have different host ranges, mortality rates, morbidity rates, and patterns of infection [3].

Influenza A viruses are further divided into highly pathogenic avian influenza (HPAI) or low pathogenic avian influenza (LPAI). Up till now, only some H5 and H7 subtypes have been confirmed as HPAI viruses. However, it is reported that some LPAI H5 and H7 subtypes can mutate to HPAI due to antigenic shift and drift phenomena [4].

Some influenza A viruses have a zoonotic potential and can cause a pandemic hazard to human population. Outbreaks of HPAI in poultry have affected the poultry industry worldwide [5]. In 2002, due to HPAI outbreaks, Chile suffered a loss of almost $31 million USD. In 2003, the HPAI outbreak resulted in the loss of more than $3387 million USD in Indonesia and $55 million USD in Vietnam. Similarly, in 2012, Mexico suffered an economic loss of approximately $475 million USD due to HPAI outbreaks [1].

2. Influenza A virus

Influenza A viruses belong to family *Orthomyxoviridae*. Influenza A viruses are single-stranded negative-sense RNA viruses having genome with 8 segmentation that encode for 10 viral proteins: hemagglutinin (HA), neuraminidase (NA), matrix proteins (M1 and M2), nucleocapsid protein (NP), nonstructural proteins (NS1 and NS2), and polymerase proteins (PB1, PB2, and PA) [6].

Influenza viruses are further classified into subtypes on the basis of their hemagglutinin (HA) and neuraminidase (NA) genes [7]. A total of 18 HA and 11 NA types has been identified up till now. On the basis of phylogenetic analysis and sequence homology of the HA gene, these viruses are clustered into virus clades [4].

A nomenclature system for influenza viruses has been established by the World Health Organization (WHO) and FAO. This system contains the type of influenza, the first place of isolation of virus, strain, and year of isolation. For example, A/ Hong Kong/156/97 would be interpreted as influenza type A, isolated in Hong Kong, strain 156, and isolated in 1997 [1].

Hemagglutinin mediates binding of the virus to sialic acid receptors at the cell surface. Neuraminidase plays its role in the detachment of the virus from the cell surface [8]. A specific type of hemagglutinin binds with a specific type of cell surface that further clarifies the difference host range for different influenza virus types [9]. Mutation of genes coding hemagglutinin and neuraminidase affects the transmission of the virus along with the alteration of the host range [10].

3. Avian influenza in birds

Healthy birds can become affected by the avian influenza virus by direct contact with an infected bird. Avian influenza virus has the capability to infect more than 100 species of birds worldwide [11]. Reservoir hosts of the virus include waterfowls and shorebirds. Low pathogenic avian influenza infection does not cause any clinical disease. But, the virus survives in the host and sometimes mutates to produce highly pathogenic avian influenza virus [12].

Some species of birds are more disease resistant than others. For example, domestic poultry is more susceptible to H5N1 HPAIV infection than wild ducks. Wild ducks spread the disease to other susceptible hosts [2].

HPAI infection in susceptible birds can cause systemic infection including damage to the nervous and circulatory system that ultimately leads to death. HPAI virus inhabits and multiplies in the respiratory and gastrointestinal tracts [13]. Clinical signs and symptoms of HPAI infection in birds include loss of appetite, diarrhea, nasal discharge, respiration problem, misshapen eggs, ataxia, and incoordination [10]. The maximum mortality rate in poultry due to HPAI infection can be up to 95%. Confirmatory diagnosis of HPAI can be done by performing PCR analysis of tracheal or fecal swabs of suspected birds [14].

4. Transmission of disease from birds

Waterfowls and shorebirds are natural reservoirs of the influenza virus, and these birds spread the virus to domestic poultry by contaminating the water source, feed, and housing of domestic poultry [15]. Influenza virus secreted in feces can survive up to 35 days at 4°C. Aerosol transmission of the virus is also possible. Indirect contamination via shoes, clothing, and contaminated feathers is also reported [2].

Interspecies transmissions of the avian influenza virus are also possible. In Europe and the United States, H1N1 and H3N2 are commonly prevalent in swine population, and outbreaks have been reported by the transmission of these viruses to susceptible turkeys and chickens [11]. In another case, an outbreak in turkey flock has been reported in Canada from a poultry worker having a respiratory problem [1].

5. Transmission of disease to humans

In most cases of human infection with the influenza virus, the previous contact with alive or dead bird was recorded. People who are involved with poultry at any level are more prone to exposure than other people [16]. Meat workers, poultry farmworkers, and bird sellers are under constant threat. Veterinarians are also at higher risk due to their contact with different types of birds [17]. Direct human to human transmission is also possible at mass gatherings such as airports, concerts, and funeral ceremonies [18].

6. Prevention and control

For the control of avian influenza in commercial and rural poultry, risk management is the most important point [18]. Implementation of good agricultural practices such as strict biosecurity measures, training of poultry workers, availability of non-contaminated water, disinfection of equipment, and decontamination of farm premises before the introduction of the new flock can decrease the chance of an outbreak of AI [16].

In case of an outbreak, rapid culling and depopulation are recommended. Rapid culling can reduce the spread of the virus and minimize economic loss [19]. Poultry and their products infected with HPAI are banned to enter the food chain in developed countries [1], whereas in developing countries, HPAI-infected meat and products are consumed as feed after cooking at high temperatures. The use of effective vaccination can limit the H5N1 HPAI virus spread [18].

7. One health perspective

The first influenza A virus pandemic in humans was recorded almost a century ago, in 1918, which resulted in the death of around 20–50 million humans worldwide [20, 21]. So far, three other pandemics of influenza A virus in humans that have caused considerable loss include the 1957 H2N2 pandemic, the 1968 H3N2 pandemic, and the 2009 H1N1 pandemic [22]. From East Asia to Southeast Asia, sporadic human infection of H5N1 viruses was reported in 2003–2004 along with outbreaks in the poultry [21].

H5N1 viruses have been reported from domesticated poultry and wild birds in Asia, North Africa, Central Africa, and Europe [23]. The transmission of HPAI H5N1 viruses from poultry to humans was first documented in 1997 in Hong Kong. Some subtypes of avian influenza virus such as H5, H7, H9, and H10 have the capability of interspecies transmission [18]. According to the World Health Organization, the total confirmed human cases of H5N1 infection to date are 860 with 454 fatal cases [24]. In 2013, a LPAI H7N9 virus caused an outbreak in China with a 36% case fatality [25]. Influenza viruses are a permanent threat for humans as well as birds.

Author details

Muhammad Abubakar[1]*, Abdullah Iqbal[2], Shumaila Manzoor[1] and Kashif Saleemi[3]

1 National Veterinary Laboratory, Islamabad, Pakistan

2 Department of Microbiology, Faculty of Biological Sciences, Quaid-i-Azam University, Islamabad, Pakistan

3 Department of Pathology, Faculty of Veterinary and Animal Sciences, University of Agriculture, Faisalabad, Pakistan

*Address all correspondence to: hayee42@yahoo.com

References

[1] Chmielewski R, Swayne DE. Avian influenza: Public health and food safety concerns. Annual Review of Food Science and Technology. 2011;**2**(1):37-57. DOI: 10.1146/annurev-food-022510-133710

[2] Beato MS, Capua I. Transboundary spread of highly pathogenic avian influenza through poultry commodities and wild birds: A review. OIE Revue Scientifique et Technique. 2011;**30**(1):51-61. DOI: 10.20506/rst.30.1.2013

[3] Shi Y, Wu Y, Zhang W, Qi J, Gao GF. Enabling the "host jump": Structural determinants of receptor-binding specificity in influenza A viruses. Nature Reviews Microbiology. 2014;**12**(12):822-831. DOI: 10.1038/nrmicro3362

[4] Lipsitch M, Barclay W, Raman R, Russell CJ, Belser JA, Cobey S, et al. Viral factors in influenza pandemic risk assessment. eLife. 2016;**5**. DOI: 10.7554/elife.18491

[5] Uyeki TM, Katz JM, Jernigan DB. Novel influenza A viruses and pandemic threats. The Lancet. 2017;**389**(10085):2172-2174. DOI: 10.1016/s0140-6736(17)31274-6

[6] Kapoor S, Dhama K. Insight into influenza viruses of animals and humans. Insight into Influenza Viruses of Animals and Humans. 2014. DOI: 10.1007/978-3-319-05512-1

[7] Antigua KJC, Choi W-S, Baek YH, Song M-S. The emergence and decennary distribution of clade 2.3.4.4 HPAI H5Nx. Microorganisms. 2019;7(6):156. DOI: 10.3390/microorganisms7060156

[8] Naguib MM, Verhagen JH, Samy A, Eriksson P, Fife M, Lundkvist Å, et al. Avian influenza viruses at the wild–domestic bird interface in Egypt. Infection Ecology and Epidemiology. 2019;**9**(1):1575687. DOI: 10.1080/20008686.2019.1575687

[9] Russell CA, Kasson PM, Donis RO, Riley S, Dunbar J, Rambaut A, et al. Improving pandemic influenza risk assessment. eLife. 2014;**3**. DOI: 10.7554/elife.03883

[10] Su S, Bi Y, Wong G, Gray GC, Gao GF, Li S. Epidemiology, evolution, and recent outbreaks of avian influenza virus in China. Journal of Virology. 2015;**89**(17):8671-8676. DOI:10.1128/jvi.01034-15

[11] Chatziprodromidou IP, Arvanitidou M, Guitian J, Apostolou T, Vantarakis G, Vantarakis A. Global avian influenza outbreaks 2010-2016: A systematic review of their distribution, avian species and virus subtype. Systematic Reviews. 2018;**7**(1):17. DOI: 10.1186/s13643-018-0691-z

[12] Yoon SW, Webby RJ, Webster RG. Evolution and ecology of influenza a viruses. Current Topics in Microbiology and Immunology. Cham: Springer; 2014. pp. 359-375

[13] Śmietanka K, Minta Z. Avian influenza in Poland. Acta Biochimica Polonica. 2014;**61**(3):453-457. DOI: 10.18388/abp.2014_1863

[14] Taubenberger JK, Morens DM. Influenza: The once and future pandemic. Public Health Reports. 2010;**125**(3 Suppl):15-26. DOI: 10.1177/00333549101250s305

[15] Short KR, Richard M, Verhagen JH, van Riel D, Schrauwen EJA, van den Brand JMA, et al. One health, multiple challenges: The inter-species transmission of influenza A virus. One Health. 2015;**1**:1-13. DOI: 10.1016/j.onehlt.2015.03.001

[16] Yoo SJ, Kwon T, Lyoo YS. Challenges of influenza A viruses in humans and animals and current animal vaccines as an effective control measure. Clinical and Experimental Vaccine Research. 2018;**7**(1):1-15. DOI: 10.7774/cevr.2018.7.1.1

[17] Myers KP, Setterquist SF, Capuano AW, Gray GC. Infection due to 3 avian influenza subtypes in united states veterinarians. Clinical Infectious Diseases. 2007;**45**(1):4-9. DOI: 10.1086/518579

[18] Neumann G, Kawaoka Y. Transmission of influenza A viruses. Virology. 2015;**479-480**:234-246. DOI: 10.1016/j.virol.2015.03.009

[19] Watanabe T, Zhong G, Russell CA, Nakajima N, Hatta M, Hanson A, et al. Circulating avian influenza viruses closely related to the 1918 virus have pandemic potential. Cell Host & Microbe. 2014;**15**(6):692-705. DOI: 10.1016/j.chom.2014.05.006

[20] Subbarao K, Matsuoka Y. The prospects and challenges of universal vaccines for influenza. Trends in Microbiology. 2013;**21**(7):350-358

[21] Neumann G, Chen H, Gao GF, Shu Y, Kawaoka Y. H5N1 influenza viruses: Outbreaks and biological properties. Cell Research. 2010;**20**(1):51-61. DOI: 10.1038/cr.2009.124

[22] Van Kerkhove MD, Mumford E, Mounts AW, Bresee J, Ly S, Bridges CB, et al. Highly pathogenic avian influenza (H5N1): Pathways of exposure at the animal-human interface, a systematic review. PLoS One. 2012;**7**(1). DOI: 10.1371/annotation/3531c496-624f-40fe-92bb-5fb3d7d1d894

[23] Chakrabarti AK, Pawar SD, Cherian SS, Koratkar SS, Jadhav SM, Pal B, et al. Characterization of the influenza A H5N1 viruses of the 2008-09 outbreaks in India reveals a third introduction and possible endemicity. PLoS One. 2009;**7**(1). DOI: 10.1371/annotation/3531c496-624f-40fe-92bb-5fb3d7d1d894

[24] WHO. Cumulative number of confirmed human cases for avian influenza A (H5N1) reported to WHO, 2003-2015. In: Epidemic Pandemic Alert Response. Geneva: WHO; 2016

[25] Li R, Bai Y, Heaney A, Kandula S, Cai J, Zhao X, et al. Inference and forecast of H7N9 influenza in China, 2013 to 2015. Eurosurveillance. 2017;**22**(7). DOI: 10.2807/1560-7917.es.2017.22.7.30462

Chapter 5

Features of Highly Pathogenic Avian Influenza (HPAI) H5N1 in Domestic Poultry

Olatunde Babatunde Akanbi, Victor Olusegun Taiwo, Emmanuel Tumininu Obishakin, Pius Stephen Ekong, Israel Joshua Barde and Clement Adebajo Meseko

Abstract

H5 and H7 subtypes are associated with the highly pathogenic form of AI (HPAI), which are extremely virulent, causing up to 100% mortality in domestic poultry. This virulence and ability to cause systemic infection have been attributed to the multibasic cleavage motif in their hemagglutinin molecule, which are recognized by subtilisin-like endoproteases that are virtually present in every tissue, making them capable of replicating in multiple tissue; hence, lesions are multisystemic (i.e., nervous, circulatory, respiratory, integumentary, musculoskeletal, hemopoietic, gastrointestinal, reproductive systems). The myriads of lesion that accompanied outbreaks of HPAI in domestic poultry as seen in Nigeria from 2006 to 2016 are as a result of the above findings. A critical look at the Nigerian HPAI situation not only revealed the general clinic-pathologic features in domestic poultry and factors that support the persistence of the virus in the environment but also gave insight to the flow of the virus in the country. A situation whereby poultry are kept in free-range, multispecies, multiage holdings with low biosecurity supports the spread of HPAI. Also, the live bird markets (LBMs) that have been fed by this unorganized poultry structure have consistently been the nidus for HPAI detection, be it in 2008 after the virus was thought to have been eradicated or in 2015, when the virus resurfaced in Lagos. It is proposed that all factors enhancing the propensity of the virus to remain in poultry should be giving the attention required. Therefore, it is important that the strict biosecurity measures that ensure prevention of HPAI incursion into poultry premises after 2008 are revamped while improving on the organization of the poultry and product supply chain in the country.

Keywords: avian influenza, multisystemic, domestic poultry, pathology, Nigeria

1. Introduction

Intensive poultry production units are an ideal viral breeding ground due to genetic homogeneity which decreases the number and variability of resistance genes resulting in little variation between individuals and therefore high infection potential for viruses [1]. Also, in the aforementioned environment, these birds do not undergo any form of reproduction; therefore, there is no coevolution with the pathogen, and this presents the conditions for the maintenance of a highly lethal

IntechOpen

strain [1]. The artificial increased density of individual host pathogens increases spread to other hosts, and the short life cycles of the virus prevent the host from developing immunity against the organism [2]. With high density and short life span, contagiousness is not under selective pressure, and a selection criteria on strains allow strains to be selected mainly on virulence, i.e., harm to the host [2]. In addition, inadequate disinfection measures between batches allow the virus to survive in the environment [2]. Three potential clinical outcomes have been observed with AI infection in birds; these are (a) no clinical signs, (b) mild disease, and (c) severe disease with death [3]. The H5 and H7 subtypes of avian influenza (AI) virus associated with HPAI, which is extremely virulent, cause up to 100% mortality in domestic poultry. The virulence and ability to cause systemic infection have been attributed to the multibasic cleavage motif (minimal consensus sequence of -R-X-K/RR-) in their hemagglutinin molecule, which are recognized by subtilisin-like endoproteases that are virtually present in every tissue of their host and preferentially expressed at the surface of respiratory and gastrointestinal epithelia [4], making them capable of replicating in multiple tissue [5, 6]; hence, lesions are multisystemic (i.e., nervous, circulatory, respiratory, integumentary, musculoskeletal, hemopoietic, gastrointestinal, reproductive systems [7]). This chapter considers avian influenza virus infection with a special X-ray on the Nigerian outbreak scenario, general clinicopathologic features in domestic poultry and factors that support the persistence of the virus in the environment, and, when not adequately controlled, how these can lead to an endemic and/or a pandemic state.

2. Avian influenza transmission

2.1 The virus

Influenza viruses are segmented negative-sense single-stranded RNA, belonging to the family *Orthomyxoviridae* [8]. This family is classified into influenza viruses' types A, B, and C, *Thogotovirus*, and *Isavirus* [9]. Only influenza type A viruses infect poultry [8], and avian influenza viruses are known to be a diverse group of viruses in the *Orthomyxoviridae* family, genus *Influenza A virus*, and have been categorized into subtypes based on the two surface glycoproteins, the hemagglutinin (H) and neuraminidase (N) [10]. There are now 18 H and 11 N surface glycoproteins [11]. Previously, HA1-16 and NA1-9 have been identified to occur naturally in avian host, mostly waterfowls where they exist in benign form (low pathogenic) [12]. Subtypes HA 17 and 18 and NA 10 and 11 were identified in bats [13] recently. Avian influenza viruses have also been further classified into two different pathotypes (low pathogenicity [LP] and high pathogenicity [HP]), based on the ability to produce disease and death in the major domestic poultry species, the chicken (*Gallus gallus domesticus*) [14]. HPAI has been shown to be caused in susceptible host species by only the avian influenza viruses of H5 and H7 subtypes, which contain multiple basic amino acids at the cleavage site of the hemagglutinin molecule, [15]. However, not all H5 and H7 avian influenza viruses are highly pathogenic. It has been shown that HPAI viruses emerge in domestic poultry from LPAI progenitors of the H5 and H7 subtypes [16–18].

2.2 Transmission

A typical flow of avian influenza virus in poultry mostly begins with the introduction of the virus to a region or country where the virus has not been known to be present. This introduction has been known to occur by way of contact of resident water fowls and/or backyard poultry with an infected migratory wild bird

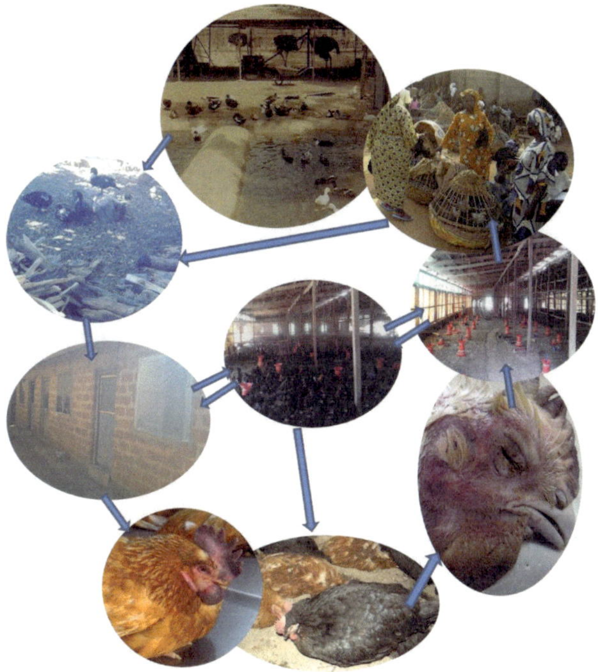

Figure 1.
A flow chart of the typical origin and transmission of avian influenza in poultry.

[19–21] which may carry any of the subtype combinations of hemagglutinin (H) and neuraminidase (N) glycoproteins. This subtype in the case of an infection with HPAI will definitely have H5 or H7 combination. This contact may occur at wetland [22, 23] areas or agroecological regions [24].

In addition, there could be direct introduction of infected bird into poultry. **Figure 1** illustrates the possibilities of the virus flow in poultry which may begin with local ducks or mixed species flock having contact (direct) with the virus by way of resident water fowls and or migratory wild birds. The virus can move by human vectors (indirect) especially when poultry attendants take care of the mixed species flock, after which a contact of free-ranging ducks and/or chickens with semi-intensive or backyard poultry may take place. At this point, the virus enters into intensive poultry directly or indirectly causing deaths.

Experience with farmers/poultry owners and attendants at the Central Diagnostic Laboratory of the National Veterinary Research Institute in Vom, Nigeria, revealed that poultry owners hurriedly sell off supposedly infected chickens to live bird and wet bird markets, from where unsuspecting public and local peasant poultry keepers buy these infected poultry for introduction into local flocks. The circle of infection can continue unabated for a very long time.

3. The Nigerian scenario

3.1 Index outbreak

Nigeria experienced an outbreak of HPAI H5N1 virus in both commercial and local poultry populations during January 2006 as an extension of the global outbreaks [7]. The index HPAI-H5N1 was confirmed in Nigeria at a commercial poultry farm in Kaduna State, and by the end of the initial outbreak, over 46,000 poultry

[25, 26] had been destroyed. This outbreak brought the Asian strain of highly pathogenic avian influenza (HPAI) H5N1 into Africa for the first time in the beginning of January 2006 [7, 27–29] in Nigeria. During this first incursion of the virus into Nigeria, the country lost excess of 1 million birds of various species [30, 31]. Since its emergence in Africa in 2006, avian influenza viruses of the H5N1 subtype have spread rapidly to poultry farms in several African countries.

This acute, generalized, fatal disease [32] affected free-ranged domestic poultry, backyard poultry, and commercial poultry comprising of chickens, ducks, geese, turkeys, guinea fowls, other gallinaceous birds, and ostriches in the poultry industry of the country. Although elsewhere in the world quails, ratites, passerine bird, flamingos, herons, raptors [32], and mammals have also been found to be susceptible to HPAI, this was not so in Nigeria. HPAI which is known to be caused by avian influenza viruses (AIVs) that are extremely virulent, resulting in up to 100% mortality in domestic chickens [33], was isolated in several outbreaks that occurred in Nigeria.

3.2 Source of the virus

Several sources have been found to be responsible for the introduction and reintroduction of the virus; these include wild bird sources, trade in poultry [29], and direct source introduction. Following the waves of outbreaks during the 2006–2007 periods, phylogeographic analysis [22] identified the north-central (Katsina, Jigawa, Yobe, Kano, Kaduna, Bauchi, and Gombe) and southwest (Lagos, Ogun, Oyo, Ekiti, and Kwara) regions as the two major sources for the HPAIV in Nigeria [22]. This supports the hypothesis that the introduction of the virus into Nigeria may be by wild birds and trade in poultry [29] and its products. Wild birds are strongly believed to be a major source of the virus to the northeastern states of Jigawa and Yobe, which are home to the Hadejia-Nguru wetlands and are said to be characterized by permanent and seasonal lakes and numerous population of migratory and residential waterfowl [22]. It is also known that this area sustains a large backyard poultry population and the highest concentration of domestic ducks, reared under free-range conditions, providing opportunities for contact between wild birds and backyard poultry [24].

3.3 The poultry structure

The poultry structure in Nigeria is comprised of two major systems, rural poultry production and commercial poultry production [34], as classified by the Food and Agricultural Organization (FAO) of the United Nation (UN). In the rural poultry production, it is a common practice to keep poultry in free-range, multispecies, multiage holdings with low biosecurity levels, thus exposing them to many at-risk contacts, and they could act as the epidemiologic link between the wild reservoir of AI viruses [22, 35] and industrial poultry. The commercial poultry production can be fully intensive or semi-intensive, depending on the level of automation and husbandry. **Figure 2A–D**, gives an insight to the poultry structure practiced in Nigeria.

3.4 Surveillance and outbreaks investigation

As far back as early February 2004, the veterinarians have been saddled with the responsibility of gearing efforts toward managing HPAIV outbreaks [37] if Nigeria was at risk or eventually experience an outbreak. Prevention strategy document for the emergency preparedness and response plan (EPP) [37] was ready as early as 2005. This included a risk analysis of the 24 wetlands in Nigeria and the two major

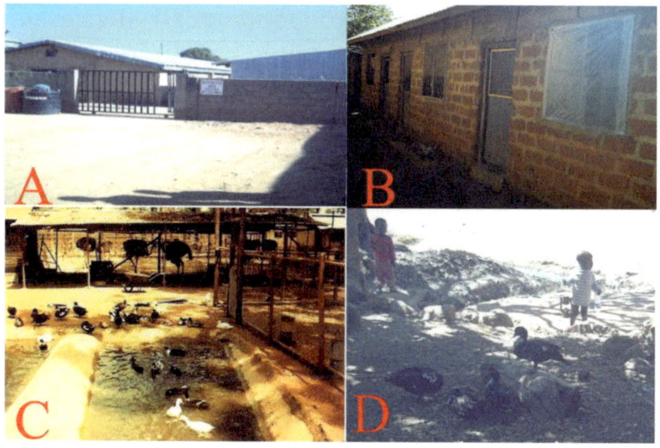

Figure 2.
(A) Intensive poultry production system in the tropics [36]. (B) A semi-intensive poultry production system in the tropics [36]. (C) A mixed species backyard poultry production system comprising of ostriches, geese, Muscovy, mallard, and Pekin ducks before the introduction of HPAI [36]. (D) An extensively (free-ranging) reared Muscovy/mallard duck flock [36].

migratory routes of wild birds, evaluation and upgrading of veterinary services, ban on importation of poultry and poultry products, and increased surveillance for the virus [37]. Surveillance and disease reporting included passive and active surveillance and regular disease reporting. The active surveillance component involved epidemiological surveillance of network of 170 points within the country and targeted surveillance of wetlands and farms [37]. Surveillance was carried out between September and November 2005 at the Nguru-Hadejia wetlands [37]. Similarly, active surveillance was carried out in the same period in the high-risk agroecological farming areas and among live bird (poultry) markets, but all these surveillance activities failed to detect H5 or H7 avian influenza virus [37]. Several investigations have been carried out and are available to the public about the HPAI H5N1 outbreaks in Nigeria, including the virological identification and confirmation [26, 28, 37, 38], epidemiology and pathology of early [7] and resurgent outbreaks [39], and molecular characterization [29], including regional mortality and morbidity characteristics [40].

3.5 Reintroduction of the virus into domestic poultry

Reintroduction of the virus to Nigeria was first detected in January 2015, when the National Veterinary Research Institute (NVRI), Vom, Nigeria, received some chicken carcasses from the Kano State Ministry of Agriculture [39]. The carcasses were gotten from a backyard-commercial poultry farm and also from a live bird market (LBM) in Kauna and Sabon Gari, Kano State, northwestern Nigeria, respectively. The farm husbandry was mixed poultry species system where different types of chickens of various ages and stages were kept and were experiencing high mortality of 350 birds daily with eventual 100% mortality observed in the older birds (54 weeks) [39]. Also, in a concurrent incidence, unusual high mortality of birds brought from the northern part of Nigeria to two LBMs in Onipanu and Mushin, Lagos State, Southwestern Nigeria, was reported [39]. The specimens were analyzed by RT-PCR and virus isolation in embryonating chicken eggs, and all samples were found to be positive for HPAI (H5N1) subtype [39]. This ended the 9-year silence of the activity of the virus in Nigerian poultry [39]. Again, a strong genetic link between viruses isolated in Nigerian poultry and wild bird from Europe has been established [21, 22, 41, 42], thereby suggesting that wild birds are the major possible source of introduction and reintroduction of HPAI viruses into Nigeria's poultry. On the other hand, rural poultry mainly kept in free-range, multispecies, multiage holdings with low biosecurity levels are exposed to many at-risk contacts and therefore act as the epidemiologic link between the wild reservoir of AI viruses and industrial poultry [22, 35]. The predominant species in the rural poultry sector of Africa is the scavenging indigenous domestic fowl (*Gallus gallus domesticus*) [43], which in most African countries has no regular health control program, may or may not have shelter, and scavenges for most of their nutritional needs [43]. In fact, village chickens have been reported to act as potential reservoirs and carriers of infections to themselves and to the more susceptible exotic breeds in commercial poultry farms [44].

3.6 Factors supporting occurrence of outbreaks

Following initial introduction of the virus from a possible migratory wild bird [22] or water fowl [20] through direct means into commercial poultry or by resident water fowls and ducks that form bridges of virus transmission from migratory wild birds [35], the virus is further spread by inadequate farm biosecurity, trade in poultry, human and vehicular exchanges between farms, and uncontrolled farm visits by poultry and poultry product vendors. Live bird markets have also been shown to harbor [39] and transmit the virus among birds and finally to household poultry upon introduction of poultry bought from live bird markets [20]. Mixed-species poultry farming has been shown to have higher odds of HPAI virus infection [39] and could harbor apparently healthy but infected duck species which may transmit the virus to susceptible chickens and turkeys. In a study conducted during the first introduction of HPAI into Nigeria, it was shown that mortality rate was much higher in mixed species flocks ($P < 0.0001$) and ranged from 4.92 to 73.15% with the chicken-duck-turkey mixed flock farms having the highest rate (73.15%) [39]. Also, it was established that higher risk of HPAI disease occurred in multiple, mixed species poultry than in single species poultry production [39]. **Figure 3** depicts a typical live bird scenario.

3.7 Control measures

Enforcement of movement control, surveillance (active and passive), and prompt payment of the revised compensation to the affected farmers, including reorganization of the LBMs which led to the successes recorded during the

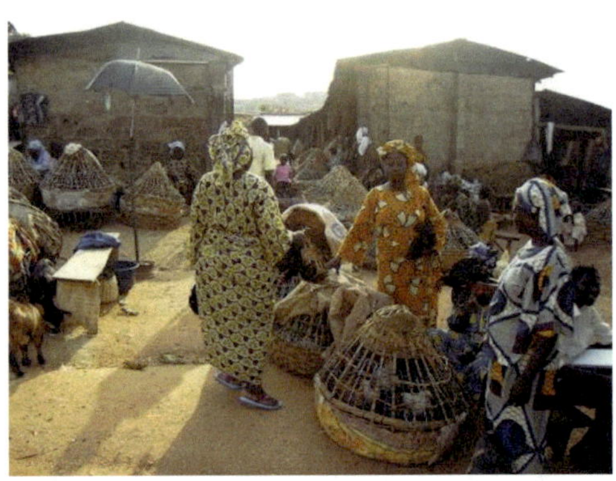

Figure 3.
A typical live bird market where poultry from different origins are sold. ©Prof. T. U Obi, University of Ilorin.

2006–2007 epizootics [45], is necessary to control HPAI in Nigeria. In these current HPAI epizootics, it has been observed that coordination and other instituted control measures, including biosecurity and compensation of affected farmers, seem to be less rigorous, and this may explain the rapid spread from the index cases to 25 states of the federation as of March 2016 [42].

4. Clinicopathologic features of avian influenza infection in domestic commercial and rural poultry: chickens and ducks

4.1 General outcome of disease

Three possible clinical outcomes have been shown to occur with AI infection in birds: there may be no clinical signs, it may result in a mild disease, and severe disease with death may occur [3]. Virus replication within the cell, tissue, organ, or a combination results in pathobiological changes which are abnormal physiological and anatomic changes. Therefore, in general, as virus replication titers increase, so do the severity of pathobiological changes such as gross and microscopic lesions with the most pathogenic virus strains causing major cell damage and death if it is sufficiently severe to affect critical organs [3] **Figure 4**.

4.2 Clinical signs

In gallinaceous domestic poultry, infection with HPAI viruses produces severe depression, severe decrease in feed and water consumption, high morbidity and mortality rates, sudden death, and occasionally nervous signs if they survive the peracute syndrome. However, the frequency of clinical signs and gross lesions varies with virus and species of bird and is not consistent in all birds [3] (**Figure 5**).

4.2.1 Chickens

Individual birds are listless and exhibit edema; cyanosis of the comb, wattles, and legs; and diarrhea. Sudden deaths without any symptoms may also occur. Signs observed and reported are sudden death, high mortality, weakness, and

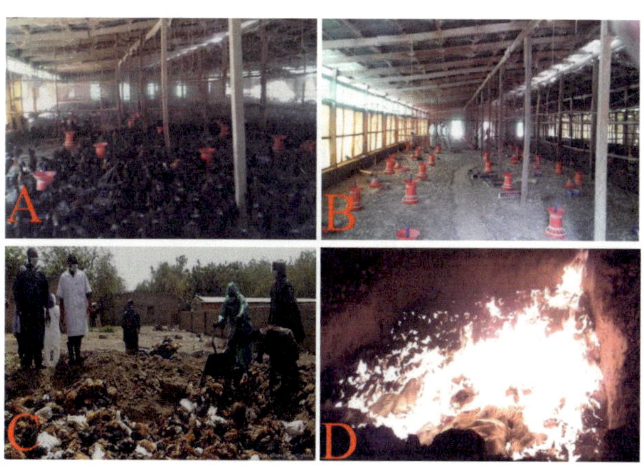

Figure 4.
(A) An open-sided layer chicken pen infected with highly pathogenic avian influenza virus. (B) The flock in A when the pen was already depopulated. (C) The poultry birds been placed in an open dug pit after depopulation. (D) The flock in A been burnt after depopulation. A and B courtesy of Dr. Luka Pam; C and D received anonymously.

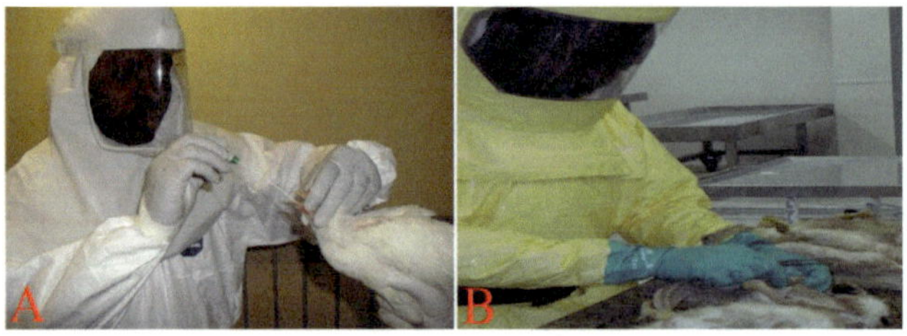

Figure 5.
(A) Testing for influenza virus using oropharyngeal swab stick. (B) Examining suspected outbreak of influenza virus infection in poultry.

recumbency. Others ranged from nasal discharges, dyspnea, coughing, sneezing, shank hyperemia and hemorrhage, inability to stand, ataxia, and torticollis. In layers, egg structural abnormalities such as shell-less egg, white-colored eggs, and soft eggs were reported.

4.2.2 Backyard poultry

In backyard poultry, sudden death is most common especially in turkeys, ducks, guinea fowls, and local chickens [31]. Signs were rarely observed and reported in these poultry species, as they were seen to die suddenly without premonitory signs although paralysis, ataxia and torticollis, dyspnea, coughing, sneezing, and diarrhea were occasionally seen and reported [31].

4.2.3 Ducks

Less vulnerable poultry species such as ducks, geese, ratites, and pigeons typically exhibit nervous symptoms including ataxia, torticollis, and seizures [46, 47].

4.3 Pathologic lesions

The frequency of gross lesions is also dependent on virus and species of bird and is not consistent in all birds [3].

4.3.1 Chickens

The main clinical and pathologic findings of HPAI are usually observed in the nervous, circulatory, respiratory, integumentary, musculoskeletal, gastrointestinal, and reproductive systems, and occasionally lesions are multisystemic. Chickens being the most frequently infected species with HPAI viruses exhibit common lesions including edema to necrosis of comb and wattle, edema of the head and legs, subcutaneous hemorrhage of legs, lungs that fill with fluid and blood, and small hemorrhages on internal organs such as the coronary fat. All of these lesions point to alternations in the cardiovascular system, which principally affects vascular endothelium and the resulting viremia. HPAI infections in gallinaceous birds have been shown to result in mortalities of up to 100% within 48 hours [48, 49]. Lesions observed in the circulatory system included congestion and cyanosis of comb and wattle, comb and wattle edema, and facial and subcutaneous edema. Within the respiratory system, there were airsacculitis and pneumonia. There was petechiation to ecchymoses of the proventricular and intestinal mucosa with resultant enteritis in the gastrointestinal system [31]. Integumentary system lesions are mainly cyanosis, edema, and ecchymotic hemorrhages, while there were inflammatory, degenerative, and necrotic lesions in the musculoskeletal system. In adult birds, mainly layers reproductive lesions were observed, and they were mainly ovarian follicular ecchymotic hemorrhages [31]. **Figure 6A–C** depicts the lesions in chickens naturally infected by HPAI virus.

4.3.2 Backyard poultry

The main pathologic findings were observed in the nervous, circulatory, respiratory, musculoskeletal, and intestinal systems, and occasionally lesions are multisystemic. Lesions observed in the circulatory system included cyanosis of comb and wattle, comb and wattle edema, and facial and subcutaneous edema. Within the respiratory system, there were nasal discharges, airsacculitis, and pneumonia [31]. Petechiation to ecchymoses of the proventricular and intestinal mucosal with resultant enteritis in the intestinal system were observed [31]. There were inflammatory, degenerative, and necrotic lesions in the musculoskeletal system [31].

4.3.3 Ducks

Ducks oftentime show one or more lesions of the circulatory system and showed nervous lesions of neuronal and Purkinje cell necrosis of the cerebrum and cerebellum [31]. There was nasal exudation, airsacculitis, and pneumonia in some ducks [31]. Enteric petechiation and ecchymoses were also observed [31] (**Figure 7**).

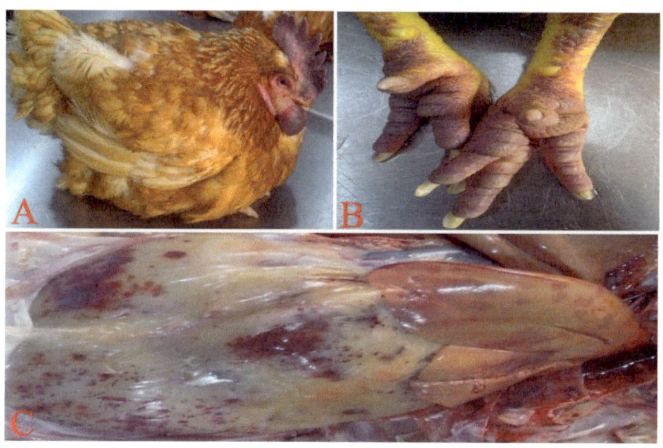

Figure 6.
(A) A layer chicken showing clinical signs of weakness and sitting on hock; the comb and wattles are congested, and the wattles are swollen. (B) The feet and shank are severely hemorrhagic. (C) The abdominal fat depot shows petechiae to ecchymotic hemorrhages which are sometimes diffuse; the liver is necrotic and friable, i.e., color is bleached and has fatty appearance.

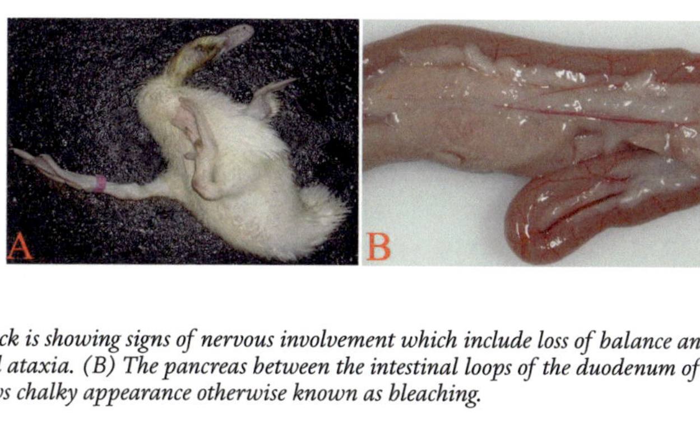

Figure 7.
(A) The Pekin duck is showing signs of nervous involvement which include loss of balance and inability to stand upright and ataxia. (B) The pancreas between the intestinal loops of the duodenum of this chicken is necrotic, i.e., shows chalky appearance otherwise known as bleaching.

5. Persistence of avian influenza viruses in poultry population

Many countries and regions have successfully controlled the virus after its occurrence, whereas some other countries face occasional reoccurrences despite intensive control efforts [50]. By the last quarter of 2007, outbreaks of HPAIV in Nigeria appeared to have been successfully controlled by measures such as "stamping out with compensation," restrictions on movement of poultry, and enhanced surveillance [19]. But the detection of new cases of HPAIV in farms from Kano and Katsina States and in apparently healthy ducks in live bird markets in Gombe and Kebbi States [19, 22, 51] proved otherwise. The viruses in sublineage H which were isolated from vultures, pigeon, guinea fowl, free-range chicken, and other birds from a wildlife park were observed to be geographically and chronologically dispersed in Nigeria following infection of the LBMs. Thus, the importance of the live bird markets in the spread of the virus in West Africa is particularly evident [52]. Also, a resurgent outbreak was recorded in January 2015, after almost 8 years following the end of the last epizootics, [39, 41]. Thus far, the outbreak has spread to several other African countries including Burkina Faso, Cote d'Ivore, Niger, Ghana, Cameroon, and Togo [42].

Influenza A viruses are known to circulate in their natural hosts and wild aquatic birds predominantly of the orders Anseriformes (ducks, geese and swans) and Charadriiformes (gulls, waders, and terns). These wild ducks are natural reservoirs of avian influenza (AI) viruses [10, 53, 54], and epidemiologic evidence and experimental infections show that domestic ducks are also susceptible to AI viruses [55, 56].

The circulation and reemergence of highly pathogenic avian influenza viruses of H5N1 subtype (HPAIV-H5N1) raise major concerns in public health and poultry industries [57]. Tens of millions of birds have died of HPAIV-H5N1 in the global poultry industry, and hundreds of millions of poultry have been slaughtered to control the spread of the virus [58]. Urgent revised control measures are required to stem waves of outbreaks and to prevent the virus from becoming enzootic in poultry if the ongoing trend of recent outbreaks in Nigeria persists, [42]. If not, this may result in severe public health consequences, as observed in countries where the virus has become enzootic in poultry [59]. In a little over a year of the reported resurgent into Nigeria, several waves of outbreaks were reported in 25 states including the Federal Capital Territory (Abuja) [42].

6. Endemic situation

Following the detection and reporting of highly pathogenic avian influenza (HPAI) H5N1 virus (clade 2.2) in Nigeria in 2006 [28] and subsequently in other parts of Africa, 11 countries in the region had reported outbreaks in poultry within a few months of its detection and eventually became enzootic in Egypt's poultry [60] causing human deaths. By July 2016, the human cases as a result of infection with HPAI H5N1 in Djibouti, Nigeria, and Egypt stand at 1, 1, and 354 people, respectively, with Egypt having the second highest number of human deaths among countries with H5N1 infections in the world [61]. The exposure of humans at the human-animal interface enzootic circulation of highly pathogenic avian influenza virus (HPAIV) in agricultural scenarios poses one of the greatest public health concerns [41]. The only human case in Nigeria, which was officially reported by the World Health Organization on February 3, 2007, was diagnosed following a thorough investigation of a fever complicated by respiratory distress which finally led to death of an average aged woman [38].

Some of the factors identified to aid the spread of the virus and enzootic situation include indiscriminate disposal of infected poultry carcasses, poor biosecurity measures and disregard for perimeter fencing, uncoordinated movement of poultry and poultry products, porous borders which aid poultry smuggling, uncontrolled and unregulated live bird market structures and activities, and indiscriminate importation of poultry and its products. These are some of the factors responsible for the transmission and spread of the 2015 H5N1 outbreak [39].

In Nigeria, the continuous interfaces of wild migratory birds with backyard flocks and subsequent movement of live birds from one state to another are strongly suspected to be the source of the virus reintroduction for the second time.

Therefore, to effectively control HPAI in Nigeria and to prevent future outbreaks and rapid spread of the virus, the continuous interfaces of wild migratory birds with backyard flocks must be taking into cognizance. Also, cluster farming and live bird market chain needs to be organized, as well as preventing in between farm transmission. In addition, it has been suggested that minimizing contacts between commercial/free-range chickens and wild birds in the northern part of Nigeria may help to avert future outbreaks [19]. Also, previous study has shown that there is a higher risk of HPAI disease occurrence in mixed poultry farming. A more prognostic approach and pragmatic plan is required for the prevention and control of HPAI in Nigeria with this resurgence, in order to elude a likely endemicity of the disease [62].

7. Conclusions

The H5 and H7 subtypes associated with the highly pathogenic form of AI (HPAI), an extremely virulent virus which causes up to 100% mortality in domestic poultry, need special efforts to ensure eradication. Bearing in mind that the intensive poultry production units are an ideal viral breeding ground for these forms of AI, all factors that enhance this propensity should be giving the attention required. A critical look at the Nigerian HPAI situation not only revealed the general clinicopathologic features in domestic poultry and factors that support the persistence of the virus in the environment but also gave insight to the flow of the virus in the country. A situation whereby poultry are kept in free-range, multispecies, multiage holdings with low biosecurity supports the spread of HPAI. Also, the LBMs that have been fed by this unorganized poultry structure have consistently been the nidus for HPAI detection, be it in 2008 after the virus was thought to have been eradicated or in 2015, when the virus resurfaced in Kano and Lagos. It is therefore important that the strict biosecurity measures that ensure prevention of HPAI incursion into poultry premises after 2008 are revamped while improving on the organization of the poultry and product supply chain in the country.

Disclosure of potential conflicts of interest

The author declared that there is no conflict of interest (financial or nonfinancial).

Abbreviations

CDC	Center for Disease Control
AI	Avian influenza

LP	Low pathogenic
HP	High pathogenic
H	Hemagglutinin
N	Neuraminidase
HA	Hemagglutinin
NA	Neuraminidase
HPAI	Highly pathogenic avian influenza
HPAIV	Highly pathogenic avian influenza virus
LBMs	Live bird markets
UN	United Nation
FAO	Food and Agriculture Organization
WHO	World Health Organization
H5N1	Hemagglutinin 5 neuraminidase 1
NVRI	National Veterinary Research Institute
EPP	Emergency preparedness and response plan

Author details

Olatunde Babatunde Akanbi[1*], Victor Olusegun Taiwo[2], Emmanuel Tumininu Obishakin[3], Pius Stephen Ekong[4], Israel Joshua Barde[5] and Clement Adebajo Meseko[6]

1 Department of Veterinary Pathology, Faculty of Veterinary Medicine, University of Ilorin, Nigeria

2 Department of Veterinary Pathology, Faculty of Veterinary Medicine, University of Ibadan, Nigeria

3 Department of Biotechnology, National Veterinary Research Institute, P.M.B. 1, Vom, Plateau State, Nigeria

4 Department of Epidemiology, National Veterinary Research Institute, P.M.B. 1, Vom, Plateau State, Nigeria

5 Laboratory of Central Diagnostic, National Veterinary Research Institute, P.M.B. 1, Vom, Plateau State, Nigeria

6 Division of Animal Influenza, Infectious and Transboundary Animal Diseases, National Veterinary Research Institute, P.M.B. 1, Vom, Plateau State, Nigeria

*Address all correspondence to: akanbi.ob@unilorin.edu.ng; olatunde_akanbi@yahoo.co.uk

References

[1] Caron A, Gaidet N, De Garine-Wichatitsky M, Morand S, Cameron EZ. Evolutionary biology, community ecology and avian influenza research. Infection, Genetics and Evolution. 2009;**9**:298-303

[2] Read AF, Taylor LH. The ecology of genetically diverse infections. Science. 2001;**292**:1099-1102

[3] Swayne DE. Understanding the complex pathobiology of high pathogenicity avian influenza viruses in birds. Avian Diseases. 2007;**51**:242-249

[4] Donata K, Globig A, Beer M. (Highly pathogenic) avian influenza as a zoonotic agent. Veterinary Microbiology. 2010;**140**:237-245

[5] Horimoto T, Nakayama K, Smeekens SP, Kawaoka Y. Proprotein-processing endoproteases PC6 and furin both activate hemagglutinin of virulent avian influenza viruses. Journal of Virology. 1994;**68**:6074-6078

[6] Rott R, Klenk HD, Nagai Y, Tashiro M. Influenza viruses, cell enzymes, and pathogenicity. American Journal of Respiratory and Critical Care Medicine. 1995;**152**:16-19

[7] Akanbi BO, Teifke JP, Ekong PS, Ighodalo ET, Ogunsan EA, Makinde AA. The epidemiology, pathology and immunohistochemistry of Nigerian highly pathogenic avian influenza (HPAI) H5N1 virus infection in chickens. In: Proceedings of the 44th NVMA Annual Congress; 22-25 October 2007; Effurun. Delta State: NVMA; 2007. pp. 162-165

[8] Aly MM, Arafa AA, Hassan MK. Epidemiological findings of outbreaks of disease caused by highly pathogenic H5N1 avian influenza virus in poultry in Egypt during 2006. Avian Diseases. 2008;**52**:269-277

[9] Buechen-Osmond C, Dallwitz M. Towards a universal virus database progress in the ICTVdB. Archives of Virology. 1996;**141**:392-399

[10] Swayne DE, Halvorson DA. Avian influenza. In: Saif YM, Barnes HJ, Gilson JR, Fadly AM, McDougald LR, Swayne DE, editors. Diseases of Poultry. 11th ed. Iowa: Iowa State University Press; 2003. pp. 135-160

[11] Centre for Disease Control (CDC). Types of influenza viruses [Internet]. 2017. Available from: https://www.cdc.gov/flu/about/viruses/types.htm [Accessed: 6 December 2018]

[12] Alexander DJ. The epidemiology and control of avian influenza and Newcastle disease. Journal of Comparative Pathology. 1995;**112**:105-126

[13] Tong S, Zhu X, Li Y, Shi M, Zhang J, Bourgeois M, et al. New world bats harbor diverse influenza A viruses. PLoS Pathogens. 2013;**9**(10):e1003657

[14] Swayne DE, Suarez DL. Highly pathogenic avian influenza. Review of Science Technology Office International Epizootics. 2003;**19**:463-482

[15] European Community. Council directive 2005/94/EC of 20 December 2005 on community measures for the control of avian influenza and repealing directive 92/40/EEC. Official Journal of the European Commission. 2005;**10**:16-65

[16] Garcia M, Crawford JM, Latimer JW, Rivera-Cruz MVZE, Perdue ML. Heterogeneity in the hemagglutinin gene and emergence of the highly pathogenic phenotype among recent H5N2 avian influenza viruses from Mexico. The Journal of General Virology. 1996;**77**:1493-1504

[17] Senne DA, Panigrahy B, Kawaoka Y, Pearson JE, Suss J, Lipkind M, et al. Survey of the hemagglutinin (HA) cleavage site sequence of H5 and H7 avian influenza viruses: Amino acid sequence at the HA cleavage site as a marker of pathogenicity potential. Avian Diseases. 1996;**40**:425-437

[18] Perdue ML, Garcia M, Senne D, Fraire M. Virulence associated sequence duplication at the hemagglutinin cleavage site of avian influenza viruses. Virus Research. 1997;**49**:173-186

[19] Fusaro A, Nelson MI, Joannis T, Bertolotti L, Monne I, Salviato A, et al. Evolutionary dynamics of multiple sublineages of H5N1 influenza viruses in Nigeria from 2006 to 2008. Journal of Virology. 2010;**84**(7):3239-3247

[20] Meseko CA, Oladokun AT, Solomon P, Yakubu B. Detection of highly pathogenic avian influenza (H5N1) in apparently healthy ducks (*Anas sparsa*) in live bird markets, Nigeria. Nigerian Veterinary Journal. 2010;**31**:164-169

[21] Meseko CA, Ehizibolo DO, Vakuru C. Migratory waterfowls from Europe as potential source of highly pathogenic avian influenza infection to Nigeria poultry. Nigerian Veterinary Journal. 2018;**39**(1):1-15

[22] Fusaro A, Joannis T, Monne M, Salviato A, Yakubu B, Meseko C, et al. Introduction into Nigeria of a distinct genotype of avian influenza virus (H5N1). Emerging Infectious Diseases. 2009;**15**(3):445-447

[23] Monne I, Joannis TM, Fusaro A, et al. Reassortant avian influenza virus (H5N1) in poultry, Nigeria. Emerging Infectious Diseases. 2008;**14**(4):637-640

[24] Cecchi G, Ilemobade A, Le Brun Y, Hogerwerf L, Slingenbergh J. Agro-ecological features of the introduction and spread of the highly pathogenic avian influenza (HPAI) H5N1 in northern Nigeria. Geospatial Health. 2008;**3**:7-16

[25] NVRI Records. Case Database. Vom, Nigeria: National Veterinary Research Institute; 2006

[26] Adene DF, Wakawa AM, Abdu PA, Lombin LH, Kazeem HM, Saidu L, et al. Clinico-pathological and husbandry features associated with the maiden diagnosis of avian influenza in Nigeria. Nigerian Veterinary Journal. 2006;**1**:32-38

[27] Enserink M. Avian influenza—H5N1 moves into Africa, European Union, and deepening global crisis. Science. 2006;**311**:932-932

[28] Joannis T, Lombin LH, De Benedictis P, Cattoli G, Capua I. Confirmation of H5N1 avian influenza in Africa. The Veterinary Record. 2006;**158**:309-310

[29] Ducatez MF, Olinger CM, Owoade AA, Tarnagda Z, Tahita MC, Sow A, et al. Molecular and antigenic evolution and geographical spread of H5N1 highly pathogenic avian influenza viruses in western Africa. Journal of General Virology. 2007;**88**:2297-2306

[30] Akanbi OB, Taiwo VO. Mortality and pathology associated with highly pathogenic avian influenza H5N1 outbreaks in commercial poultry production systems in Nigeria. International Scholarly Research Notices. 2014:1-7. DOI: 10.1155/2014/415418. Article ID: 415418

[31] Akanbi OB, Taiwo VO. Backyard poultry mortality associated with highly pathogenic avian influenza (HPAI) H5N1 outbreaks in Nigeria. IOSR Journal of Agriculture and Veterinary Science. 2014b;7(9):23-27

[32] Klopfleisch R, Werner O, Mundt E, Harder T, Teifke JP. Neurotropism of highly pathogenic avian influenza virus

A/chicken/Indonesia/2003 (H5N1) in experimentally infected pigeons (*Columba livia* f. domestica). Veterinary Pathology. 2006;**43**:463-470

[33] Muzaffar SB, Takekawa JY, Prosser DJ, Newman SH, Xiao X. Rice production systems and avian influenza: Interactions between mixed-farming systems, poultry and wildbirds. Waterbirds. 2010;**33**(1):219-230

[34] Adene DF, Oguntade AE. The Structure and Importance of the Commercial and Village Based Poultry Industry in Nigeria. 1st ed. Rome: Food and Agricultural Organization; 2006

[35] Cecchinato M, Comin A, Bonfanti L, Terregino C, Monne I, Lorenzetto M, et al. Epidemiology and control of low pathogenicity avian influenza infections in rural poultry in Italy. Avian Diseases. 2011;**55**:13-20

[36] Akanbi OB, Taiwo VO. Husbandry practices and outbreak features of natural highly pathogenic avian influenza (H5N1) in Turkey flocks in Nigeria, 2006-2008. Journal of World's Poultry Research. 2015;**5**(4):109-114

[37] Maina JA. Current status of highly pathogenic avian influenza (HPAI) in Nigeria. In: Proceeding of the 4th International Conference on Avian Influenza; 6-8 December 2006; Bamako, Mali; 2006

[38] Joannis TM, Meseko CA, Oladokun AT, Ularamu HG, Egbuji AN, Solomon P, et al. Serologic and virologic surveillance of avian influenza in Nigeria, 2006-7. Eurosurveillance. 2008;**13**(42):1-5

[39] Akanbi OB, Meseko CA, Odita CI, Shittu I, Rimfa AG, Ugbe D, et al. Epidemiology and clinicopathological manifestation of resurgent highly pathogenic avian influenza (H5N1) virus in Nigeria, 2015. Nigerian Veterinary Journal. 2016;**37**(3):175-186

[40] Saidu L, Wakawa AM, Abdu PA, Adene DF, Kazeem HM, Ladan KC, et al. Impact of avian influenza in some states of Nigeria. International Journal of Poultry Science. 2008;**7**(9):913-916

[41] Monne I et al. Highly pathogenic avian influenza (H5N1) virus in poultry, Nigeria. Emerging Infectious Diseases. 2015;**21**(7):1275-1277

[42] Shittu I, Meseko CA, Gado DA, Olawuyi AK, Chinyere CN, Anefu E, et al. Highly pathogenic avian influenza (H5N1) in Nigeria in 2015: Evidence of widespread circulation of WA2 clade 2.3.2.1c. Archives of Virology. 2017;**162**:841-847

[43] Kitalyi A. FAO Inter-Departmental Working Group on Poultry. Rome, Italy: Food and Agricultural Organization of the United Nations; 1998

[44] Adu FD, Edo U, Sokale B. Newcastle disease: The immunological status of Nigerian local chickens. Tropical Veterinarian. 1986;**4**:149-152

[45] Oladokun AT, Meseko CA, Ighodalo E, et al. Effect of intervention on the control of highly pathogenic avian influenza in Nigeria. The Pan African Medical Journal. 2012, 2012;**13**:14. DOI: 10.11604/pamj.2012

[46] Kwon YK, Joh SJ, Kim MC, Sung HW, Lee YJ, Choi JG, et al. Highly pathogenic avian influenza (H5N1) in the commercial domestic ducks of South Korea. Avian Pathology. 2005;**34**:367-370

[47] Werner O, Starick E, Teifke JP, Klopfleisch R, Prajitno TY, Beer M, et al. Minute excretion of highly pathogenic avian influenza virus A/chicken/Indonesia/2003 (H5N1) from experimentally infected domestic pigeons (*Columbia livia*) and lack of transmission to sentinel chickens. The Journal of General Virology. 2007;**88**:3089-3093

[48] Swayne DE. Understanding the ecology and epidemiology of avian influenza viruses: Implications for zoonotic potential. In: Brown C, Bolin CA, editors. Emerging Diseases of Animals. Washington, DC: ASM Press; 2000. pp. 101-130

[49] Perkins LEL, Swayne DE. Pathobiology of A/Chicken/Hong Kong/220/97 (H5N1) avian influenza virus in seven gallinaceous species. Veterinary Pathology. 2001;**38**:149-164

[50] Gilbert M, Xiao XM, Pfeiffer DU, Epprecht M, Boles S, Czarnecki C, et al. Mapping H5N1 highly pathogenic avian influenza risk in Southeast Asia. Proceedings of the National Academy of Sciences of the United States of America. 2008;**105**:4769-4774

[51] WHO/OIE/FAO H5N1 Evolution Working Group. Toward a unified nomenclature system for highly pathogenic avian influenza virus (H5N1). Emerging Infectious Diseases. 2008;**14**:1

[52] Fasina FO, Bisschop SPR, Joannis TM, Lombin LH, Abolnik C. Molecular characterization and epidemiology of the highly pathogenic avian influenza H5N1 in Nigeria. Epidemiology and Infection. 2008;**137**(4):456-463. DOI: 10.1017/S0950268808000988

[53] Kawaoka Y, Chambers TM, Sladen WL, Webster RG. Is the gene pool of influenza viruses in shorebirds and gulls different from that in wild ducks? Virology. 1988;**163**(1):247-250

[54] Stallknecht DE. Ecology and epidemiology of avian influenza viruses in wild bird populations: Waterfowl, shorebirds, pelicans, cormorants. In: Proceedings of the Fourth International Symposium on Avian Influenza; 1998. pp. 61-69

[55] Chen H, Deng G, Li Z, Tian G, Li Y, Jiao P, et al. The evolution of H5N1 influenza viruses in ducks in southern China. Proceedings of the National Academy of Sciences of the United States of America. 2004;**101**:10452-10457

[56] Shortridge KF, Zhou NN, Guan Y, Gao P, Ito T, Kawaoka Y, et al. Characterization of avian H5N1 influenza viruses from poultry in Hong Kong. Virology. 1998;**252**(2):331-342

[57] Capua I, Alexander D. Perspectives on the global threat: The challenge of avian influenza viruses for the world's veterinary community. Avian Diseases. 2010;**54**:176-178

[58] Iwami S, Takeuchi Y, Liu X. Avian flu pandemic: Can we prevent it? Journal of Theoretical Biology. 2009;**257**:181-190

[59] Abdelwhab EM, Hassan MK, Abdel-Moneim AS, et al. Introduction and enzootic of A/H5N1 in Egypt: Virus evolution, pathogenicity and vaccine efficacy ten years on. Infection, Genetics and Evolution. 2016;**40**:80-90. DOI: 10.1016/j.meegid.2016.02.023

[60] FAO. H5N1 HPAI spread in Nigeria and Increased risk for Neighboring countries in West Africa [Internet]. 2015. Empres Watch, Vol. 32. Available from: http://www.fao.org/3/a-i4561e.pdf [Accessed: 20 May 2016]

[61] World Health Organization. Cumulative number of confirmed human cases for avian influenza A(H5N1) reported to WHO, 2003-2015 [Internet]. 2016. Available from: http://www.who.int/influenza/human_animal_interface/Influenza_Summary_IRA_HA_interface_07_19_2016.pdf?ua=1 [Accessed 29 July 2016]

[62] Ifende VI, Meseko CA, Odita CI, Akanbi BO, Moses GD, James AS, et al. Highly pathogenic avian influenza in Nigeria: Overview of 2015 outbreaks. In: NVRI Seminar Series Volume 2015; 5 November 2015; Vom, Nigeria; 2015. pp 147-152

Chapter 6

The Thrift of Avian Influenza in Indonesia

Khrisdiana Putri, Sitarina Widyarini, Sugiyono and Widya Asmara

Abstract

The circulating H5N1 Highly Pathogenic Avian Influenza in chicken has created devastating problems in Indonesia since 2003. Although human cases of Avian Influenza could be exceptionally reduced, however, it remains unsettled in poultry. Phylogenetic analysis of H5N1 virus (2003–2011) revealed the introduction of a single ancestral of 2.1 HA clade before 2003. The enzootic clade subsequently evolved into fourth order with predominantly 2.1.3.2. Pathological lesions showed cyanotic wattle, torticollis and haemorrhage in chicken feet and multi-internal organs. However, the introduction of vaccination and stringent biosecurity resulted in milder manifestations compared to classical lesions. In 2012, unusual high mortality in duck farms revealed the introduction of exotic clade 2.3.2.1. Despite the inefficient transmission of avian virus to humans and experimental receptor binding of 2.3.2.1 virus that showed avian preference, substitution of N158D and E190D in HA gene indicates possible threat to humans. In the same year, the Government of Indonesia announced the introduction of H9N2. Furthermore, a recent publication (2018) has reported new reassortant between HPAIV H5N1 and LPAIV H3N8 with resulting virulence attenuation in chicken.

Keywords: chicken, Indonesia, antigenic thrift, pathological lesion

1. Introduction

Avian Influenza (AI) is influenza A virus of avian origin, which may cause disease in domestic and wild birds and in some cases can infect mammalian species, including humans. The highly pathogenic variant (HPAI) has spread to more than 60 countries in Africa, Asia, Australia, Europe and North and South America only within decades. The disease has continuously involved in detrimental impact to poultry farms despite global efforts towards control and eradication. The Indonesian lineage has attracted human health community for its zoonotic attribute by demonstrating the capacity for causing three family cluster cases (West Java, Banten and North Sumatera) with one of them being the largest case in human AI history [1–3]. However, surveillance of H5N1 antibody in poultry farmers from human H5N1 outbreak areas was reported and not detected [4].

Molecular identification on samples obtained during surveillance for H5N1 virus in municipal of Muntilan, Center Java, conducted by Regional Influenza Working Group, after suspected human H5N1 infection announced in 2005, were able to identify H5N1 virus in pet animals and fish pond in the housing areas. However, virus

IntechOpen

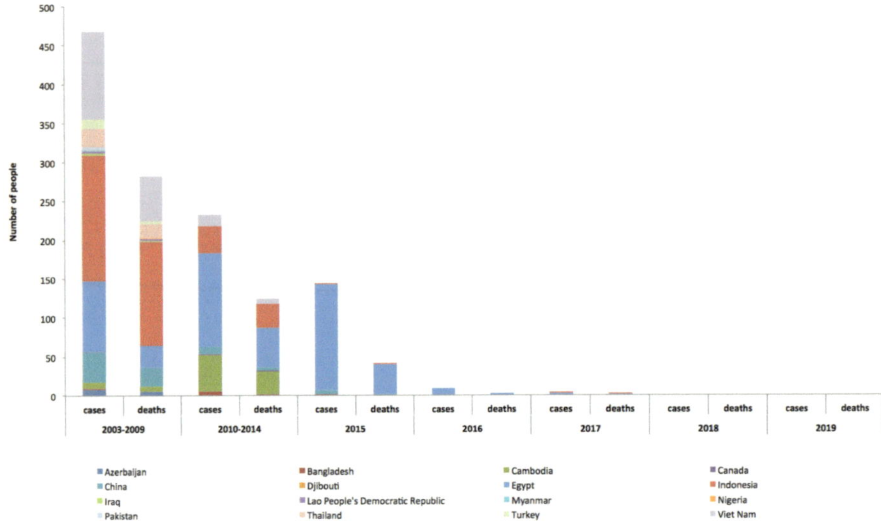

Figure 1.
Number of human Avian Influenza A (H5N1) cases by reporting country and month of onset (Taken from the World Health Organisation. Influenza at human-animal interface. Summary and assessment as of 1 May 2015 https://www.who.int/influenza/human_animal_interface/Influenza_Summary_IRA_HA_interface_1_May_2015.pdf).

sequences are not available. The number of human deaths in Indonesia were outgrowing to 150 by 2011 (**Figure 1**) [2, 5–7] with 46% reported to have direct contact with infected poultry [7]. Although, to date the virus demonstrated inefficient person-to-person transmission, ongoing outbreaks in poultry pose warning to possibly establish human reassortant Avian Influenza virus [8]. New outbreaks of H5N1 in 2014 in Cambodia, China, India, Korea, Lybia, Russia and Vietnam have shown high adaptability in a heterogeneous ecosystem, requiring urgent need for reliable surveillance tool to improved strategies to control and eradicate this enzootic disease.

2. Host specificity of Asian lineage virus

Part of the HA protein that binds to the host receptor [called the receptor binding site (RBS)] has a unique amino acid arrangement which contributes to viral specificity to the host [9].

Infection occurs when the viral ligand binds to a glycoprotein or glycolipid receptors on the cell surface possessing sialylgalactose terminal group [Neu5Ac (α2-3) Gal] or [Neu5Ac (α2-6) Gal]. Influenza virus of 226Gln and 228Gly avian origin prefers to bind to [Neu5Ac (α2-3) Gal], while influenza virus of 226Leu and 228Ser human origin binds specifically to [Neu5Ac (α2-6) Gal] [9, 10]. The fact the epithelial cells of human respiratory tract mainly contain [Neu5Ac (α2-6) Gal], while the majority in chicken is [Neu5Ac (α2-3) Gal], has provided an explanation the avian origin virus cannot readily infect humans. The shift in host specificity is possible due to the changes in amino acids in RBS through genetic mutations. Experimentally substituting an amino acid of Ser228Gly in addition to Leu226Gln of human origin virus has supported viral replication in duck intestines [11]. Although, solely mutation event of single amino acid in RBS was adequately altering binding specificity to the receptor [12, 13]. Amino acid substitution Ser227Asn in highly pathogenic avian influenza virus (HPAIV) H5N1 of Asia strain decreases its affinity for the receptor [Neu5Ac (α2-3) Gal] and gives the virus ability to bind to [Neu5Ac (α2-6) Gal] moderately. This indicates that mutations in RBS are capable to induce cross-species transmission without genetic reassortment [14].

A genetic rearrangement between influenza viruses of avian origin and influenza viruses from mammals has the potential to emerge new pandemic influenza virus strains in humans. Classical genetic reassortment model has settled pigs as mixing vessel to both viruses. The basis of the model is the specificity of the influenza virus strain to the host cell surface receptors [15, 16].

The emergence of four influenza pandemics, 1918 (H1N1), 1957 (H2N2), 1968 (H3N2), and 1977 (H1N1) was not due to genetic reassortment in pigs. The specificities of the receptors in haemagglutinin gene of 1918 virus vary between strains. Isolates A/South Caroline/1/18 tend to bind to [Neu5Ac (α2-6) Gal] receptors, while isolates A/New York/1/18 have the ability to bind both [Neu5Ac (α2-6) Gal] and [Neu5Ac (α2-3) Gal] receptors. Compared to the H1 virus from avian origin in general, isolates A/New York/1/18 differ only in amino acid 190. The viral HA mutation in this position from Asp to Glu decreases the ability of the virus to bind to the [Neu5Ac (α2-6) Gal] receptor and increases preference to the [Neu5Ac (α2-3) Gal] (avian receptor) [13]. The avian influenza virus that caused the outbreak in Asia in 2003–2004 did not show such characteristics. Some viruses isolated from Vietnam, Thailand, Hong Kong and Indonesia, both from human and avian, show similarities in amino acid sequences in the RBS area and have a preference for binding to [Neu5Ac (α2-3) Gal] (avian receptors) [12, 17–19].

3. Indonesia situation

Highly Pathogenic Avian Influenza (HPAI) has been a major problem for poultry industry in Indonesia till today. Since first announced in 2003–2004 (**Figure 2**), H5N1 outbreak was rapidly spread to most provinces, before abated by the end of 2007, after causing death to more than 16 million poultry [2, 5, 7]. In April 2011, a new outbreak was reported from Gorontalo, leaving only one province free of disease [20].

Phylogenetic analysis of Indonesian 2.1. clade virus indicated direct precursor-descendant link to viruses of genotype Z, isolated from Hunan province, China in 2002, presumably as single introduction. However, the spread and transmission from Hunan to Indonesia remained unclear [21, 22].

Up to the year 2008, all Indonesian H5N1 viruses have been classified into clade 2.1, with three virus sublineages: 2.1.1, 2.1.2 and 2.1.3. The viruses within clade 2.1.1 were mainly isolated from HPAI-infected poultry during the outbreaks between

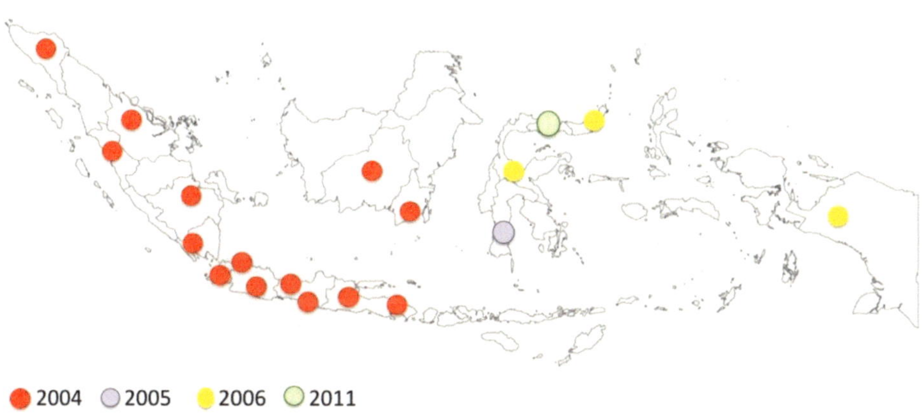

Figure 2.
H5N1 Avian Influenza poultry epidemic in Indonesia. (Map by Free Vector Maps. https://freevectormaps.com/indonesia/ID-EPS-01-0003).

2003 and 2005. The clade 2.1.2 viruses were isolated from avian- and human-derived predominantly from Sumatra between 2004 and 2007, while clade 2.1.3 viruses discovered in 2004, were isolated either from birds or from humans. Interestingly, when clade 2.1.3 viruses have begun to predominate, the numbers of clade 2.1.1 and 2.1.2 isolates were subsequently declined. Although 2.1.3 viruses have spread and become endemic in many provinces in Indonesia, a new sublineage virus has emerged since 2004. In September 2012, several duck farms from Central Java have reported high mortality of AIV H5 subtype. Interestingly, the HA genes of the duck isolates were not related to long-established Indonesian clade 2.1 isolates but closely resembled clade 2.3.2.1 viruses, which recently were found in Vietnam, China and Hong Kong [23].

Bali Island has reported only one human death because of Avian Influenza until 2017, although Bali is speculated as an ideal environment for influenza re-assortment: world-renowned tourism destination, suckling pigs, and fighting cocks tradition. Circulating A(H5N1) viruses obtained during surveillance of A(H5N1) viruses in Bali between 2009 and 2011 concluded clade 2.1 [24, 25]. Although incident of human death has occurred in Bali, the HA gene analysis at 226Q and 228G of chicken isolates yet showed binding preference to avian host. However, a single mutation finding at S137A has shown the potential of recognizing human receptor. Although evolution analysis of obtained isolates from Bali (A/Ck/Klungkung/T/2009 and A/Ck/Bali/Y/2009) is unable to determine due to lack of HA gene sequences of Indonesian isolate available in GenBank, phylogenetic analysis has clustered these isolates with the only Indonesian domestic cat virus (**Figure 3**). Consistent with the outbreak in Thailand, the HA gene of pigeon, chicken, tiger, and human isolates were closely related [26]. The potency of pigs as a mixing vessel for avian virus to adapt in human host is also unable to analyze due to the lack of available sequences in GenBank. However, the phylogenetic analysis of swine virus from Bali showed a close relation to other pig and chicken viruses within the corresponding year [27].

Surveillance of A(H5N1) viruses in live bird markets (LBM) during 2012-2013 indicated that most viruses were HPAIV (H5N1), which were related to other clade 2.1.3.2a viruses. The surveillance also detected LPAIV A (H3N8) A/environment/West Java/KRW54/2012, which forms outlier with other LPAI H3 of Eurasian lineage. The A (H3N8) also demonstrated 90% nucleotide identical to A/Duck/Siberia/100/2001. Importantly, genetic reassortment among AIV isolates is occurred by contribution of internal and NA gene segments of LPAIV virus into HPAIV (H5N1) clade 2.1.3.2a virus. Three reassortant viruses (A/Muscovy Duck/East Java/SB29/2012, A/Muscovy Duck/East Java/LM47/ 2012 and A/Ck/East Java/BP21/2012) possessed PB2, PB1 and NS genes of LPAI virus, while the surface glycoproteins (HA and NA) and other internal genes (PA, NP and M) were contribution of HPAI A(H5N1) virus lineage. The experimental data of the reassortant HPAI A(H5N1) viruses showed slight attenuation possibly due to acquisition of LPAI internal genes to HPAI virus [8]. In 2017, the government of Indonesia has officially announced the introduction of enzootic H9N2 subtype; however, it is still poorly documented. The introduction of LPAIV A(H9N2) may possess new hidden endemic zoonotic threat. Chinese Centre for Diseases Control and Prevention has highlighted the role of H9N2 as "incubators" to facilitate new zoonotic human avian strain [28].

Since 2004, the Indonesian Government have been applying vaccination in poultry to control AIV H5N1 and simultaneously intensify biosecurity in poultry farm, conducting active diseases surveillance, application of stamping-out policy limited to endemic area and extensive to newly infected area, and improving public awareness of the disease [29, 30]. Although vaccine can be used as a prevention tool, it does not provide full protection or "sterilising immunity" [31]. Vaccine application for Avian Influenza in the field is recommended to allow to serologically differentiate vaccinated birds from infected (DIVA) [32–34]. Proposed strategy for DIVA by the use of sentinel

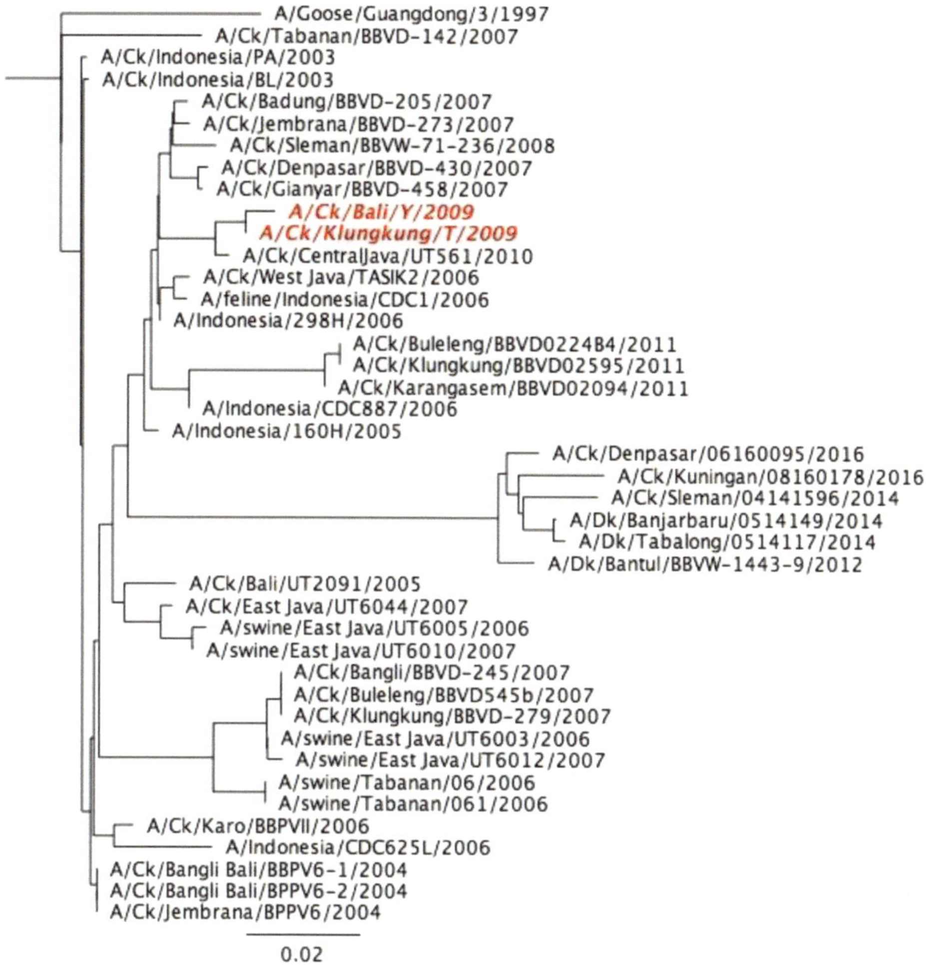

Figure 3.
Phylogenetic tree analysis of A/Ck/Klungkung/T/2009 and A/Ck/Bali/Y/2009 A (H5N1) compared to other sequences of poultry, human, swine and human Indonesia available in GenBank. A/Goose/Guangdong/1997 was served as outgroup in rooted neighbour-joining calculation. The scale indicated 0.02 nt substitution per site. The analysis was performed using Geneious R.10 (Biomatters, Ltd).

chickens has been conducted in West Java [30, 35]. However, as possible, new infections in the flock may originate from these sentinel naive birds, which may acquire infection prior to being placed; this DIVA strategy has not received widespread acceptance in Indonesia. Several alternative strategies using viral protein for marker in chickens have been developed, that is, NS1 [36, 37], M2e [38, 39] and HA2 [40, 41].

4. Pathological features

The pathological features of Avian Influenza infection in poultry since the first outbreak in Indonesia have undergone slight changes over time. The pathological changes are currently showing milder description compared to classical discovery in the middle of 2003. Avian Influenza viruses in poultry were reported to produce asymptomatic to mild upper respiratory infections, egg production loss to rapid fatal systemic disease [42].

Pathogenicity attributes of AI virus were categorised as low pathogenic avian influenza virus (LPAIV) and highly pathogenic avian influenza viruses (HPAIV) [43, 44].

The low pathogenic variant (LPAI) in poultry describes signs of respiratory diseases [43, 45], while high pathogenic variant (HPAI) demonstrates severe systemic signs with necrotic and inflammatory lesions of skin, viscera and brain [46–48], although mortality may occur in the absence of clinical signs [42]. The degree of clinical manifestations and recovery rate of the birds are notably age-related. Older birds generally recover within a week, since the onset of clinical signs. Conversely, younger birds are suffering from severe respiratory symptoms as of reflecting in high mortality rates (40–97%). Furthermore, co-infection of other secondary pathogens also contribute to high mortality [45]. Low-pathogenic infection is typically demonstrating low mortality (<5%) accompanied by high morbidity (>50%) [44, 45], contrarily, infection by HPAI virus results in 100% mortality of susceptible poultry species [43, 48].

Low pathogenic variant AI demonstrates clinically mild to severe respiratory signs, i.e., coughing, sneezing, swollen infraorbital, excessive ocular and nasal discharge [43, 44]. Infected birds, in general show lethargy, mild weight loss, neurological signs, occasional diarrhoea and sudden drop in eggs production from 30 to 80% during acute phase [43–45, 49]. In humans, a high viral load in pharynx resulted in fatality [50].

Presented clinical signs of infected birds depend on the species and age of the host, virus strain and also the pathophysiological changes in the respiratory, digestive, urinary, nervous and reproductive systems [44, 51, 52]. Hence, avian influenza virus pathobiology varies among strains and the host species. Therefore, pathobiology characters of new avian influenza virus are important to control the outbreaks and understand the epidemiology of this disease [53].

Clinical signs and pathological features of H5N1 in layer chickens from East Java, Central Java, West Java and Yogyakarta during 2003–2005 outbreaks have demonstrated depression, loss of appetite, neurologic disorder, respiratory disorder, egg production drop and diarrhoea [54]. These clinical signs were similar to previously described infections naturally or experimentally with highly pathogenic avian influenza virus in domestic poultry [44, 45, 51, 55, 56].

On post-mortem examination of infected chicken showed severe subcutaneous haemorrhages, oedema in the wattles, head, neck, and the leg shanks appeared haemorrhages [55]. However, Mutinelli et al. [45] and Elbers et al. [57] also described peritonitis; haemorrhage, enlarged and hardened of pancreas; enlarged

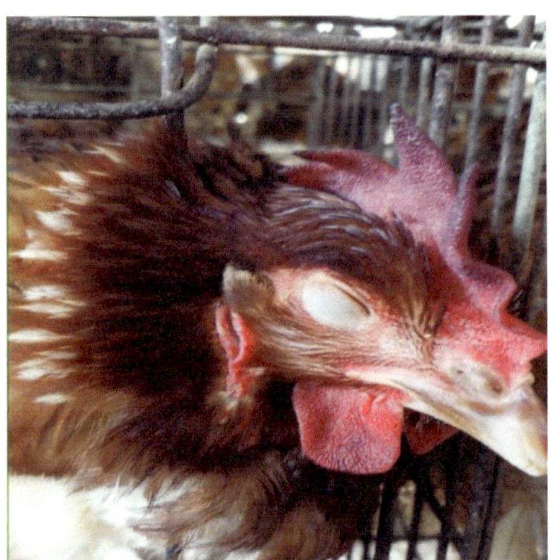

Figure 4.
Latest cases of Avian Influenza: Cyanotic wattles (Courtesy: Dr. Sitarina Widyarini).

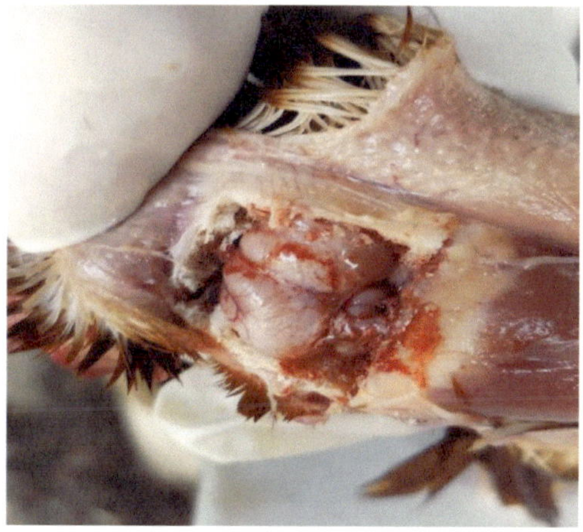

Figure 5.
Latest cases of Avian Influenza: Brain congestion (Courtesy: Dr. Sitarina Widyarini).

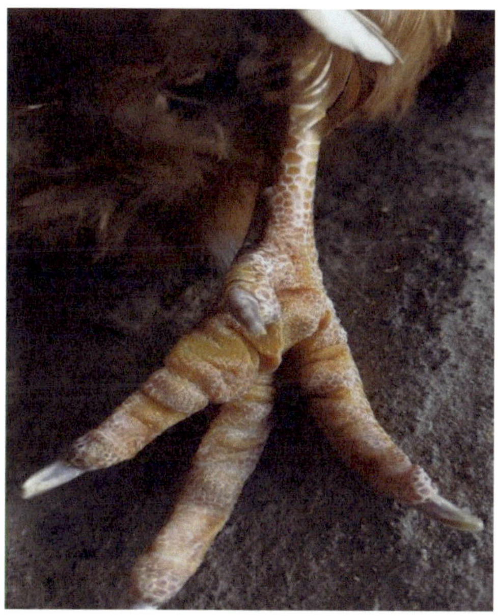

Figure 6.
Latest case of Avian Influenza: Haemorrhages feet (Courtesy: Dr. Sitarina Widyarini).

with whitish and dark brown haemorrhage of liver areas. In a few cases, proventriculus and ventriculus showed petechial haemorrhages [45, 55, 57], haemorrhages of comb and wattles, ecchymose haemorrhages in the skin of the breast and abdomen [47]. Similar lesions such as cyanotic wattles, swollen head and comb, haemorrhages in the skeletal muscles, abdominal fat, proventriculus and feet were also observed in chicken during 2003–2005 Avian Influenza outbreaks in Indonesia [54]. Furthermore, in layer chickens, haemorrhagic ovary and atrophy oviduct were also found [54, 56, 58]. Similar findings in mute and whooper swans infected by HPAI, was showing coalescent haemorrhages with necrosis in the pancreas [59, 60], kidney enlargement yet elastic without deposits of uric acid [45].

Recent case in layer chicken of 40 weeks from East Java (August, 2018) with cyanotic wattles (**Figure 4**), brain congestion (**Figure 5**), haemorrhages in the feet (**Figure 6**) and proventriculus (**Figure 7**), haemorrhages and adhesion

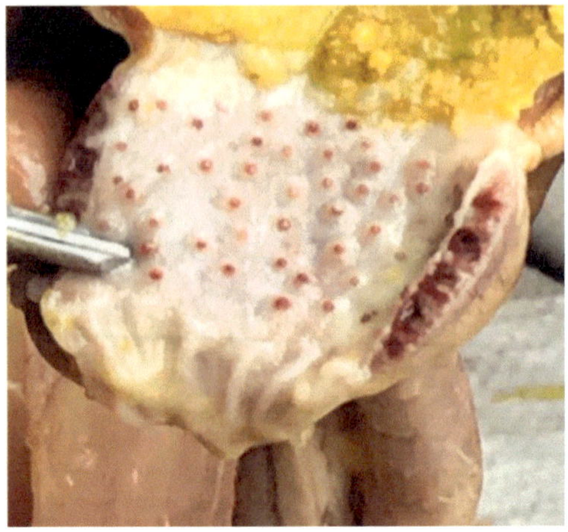

Figure 7.
Latest case of Avian Influenza: Proventriculus Haemorrhages (Courtesy: Dr. Sitarina Widyarini).

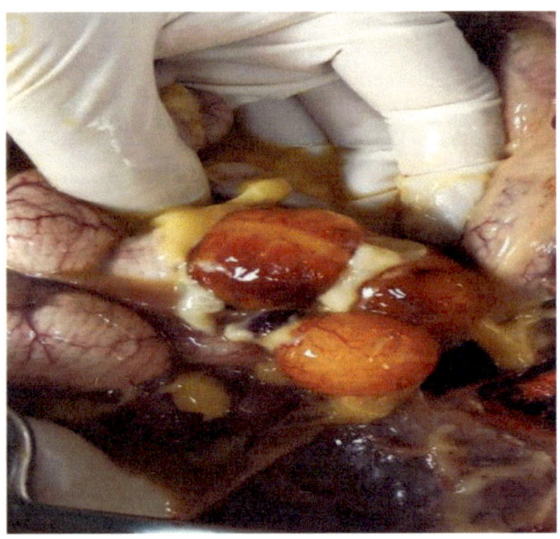

Figure 8.
Latest case of Avian Influenza: Ovarial Haemorrhages (Courtesy: Dr. Sitarina Widyarini).

between ovarian follicles (**Figure 8**), haemorrhage of abdominal fat (**Figure 9**), haemorrhage of pectoral muscles (**Figure 10**), swollen and oedematous kidney (**Figure 11**). The farm experienced 20% mortality rates within 3 weeks and the egg production dropped by 18% suddenly in 5 days. Vaccination for avian influenza H5 was done at 14 weeks of chick age. Molecular identification was confirming H5 subtype. In a few cases, virus can be isolated from properly vaccinated flock [61].

Histopathological findings of HPAIV-infected chicken and turkey were dominated by acute haemorrhages (skin, under serous membrane, mucosae and pectoral muscles), oedema (skin of head, neck, legs and lungs) and necrosis (skin, pancreas, spleen and heart) [42, 46, 49, 55, 62–66]. The comb and wattles showed markedly severe cellulitis associated with congestion, oedema and mild heterophilic infiltration in the dermis and subcutis [55]. Lymphocytic meningo-encephalitis and meningo-encephalomyelitis with multifocal gliosis, degeneration of neuron, necrosis and neuronophagia, as well as mild-to-moderate perivascular cuffs, with predominance of macrophages and lymphocytes in both grey and white matter in the majority of brain region [60, 67, 68]. Necrosis with focal lymphohistiocytic

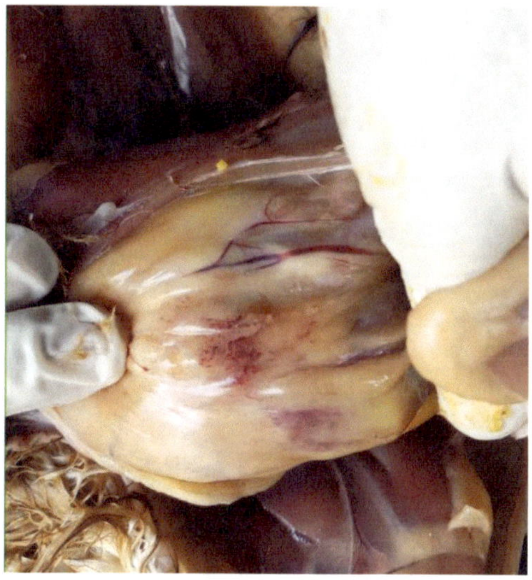

Figure 9.
Latest case of Avian Influenza: Abdominal fat haemorrhages (Courtesy: Dr. Sitarina Widyarini).

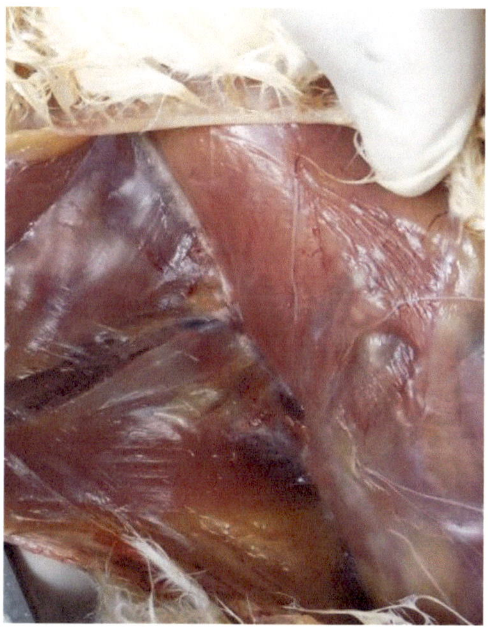

Figure 10.
Latest case of Avian Influenza: Pectoral muscles haemorrhages (Courtesy: Dr. Sitarina Widyarini).

infiltration in the myocardium, focal necrosis in the pancreas and other organs (e.g. lungs, lymphatic organs and skeletal muscles) are defined as important histopathological lesions [58, 60, 68].

Histological lesions associated with the presence of viral antigen were observed in the tissue of infected chickens. Several studies have observed intranuclear and intracytoplasmic viral antigens distribution at surrounding tissues of parenchymal myofibres and capillary endothelium of the heart, hepatocytes and sinusoidal endothelium of the liver, pulmonary endothelium, pancreas, kidney, central nervous system, leukocytes of the Peyer's patches, bursa, epithelium of the adrenal glands, renal tubules and pancreatic acini [44, 55, 69, 70].

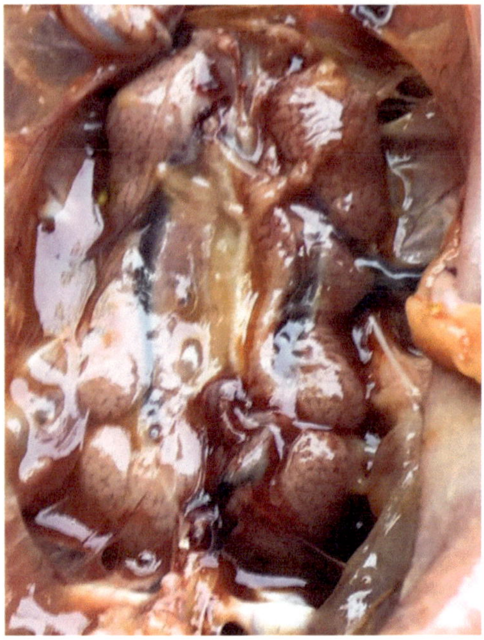

Figure 11.
Latest case of Avian Influenza: Swollen and oedematous kidney (Courtesy: Dr. Sitarina Widyarini).

5. Conclusion

Vaccine application and stringent biosecurity practices helped to suppress the viral load in the flock. As consequences, the morbidity and mortality rate is suppressed, the presentation of clinical signs is milder although the gross pathology features remained consistent. The introduction of H9N2 has initiated the new threat. Egg production drop is today mainly observed as an indication of infection regardless of the virus subtype, although as the latest published active surveillance data (2012–2013) continued blaming H5N1. The masking effect of partial low-level herd immunity may be responsible for the phenomenon.

Virus isolated from chicken with both specific and non-specific lesion between 2003 and 2006 showed high pathogenic avian influenza virus based on molecular marker analysis. Although vaccination has been applied, full viral characterisation continues, evaluation of antibody protective response after vaccination and differentiation between vaccinated and infected birds is needed. Cartography surveillance of avian virus is importantly required to understand cross-immunity of latest strains to use as vaccine seeds. Antigen panel is a must in order to predict future outbreak. Enforcement on regulation for live birds market (LBM) is a must, considering massive human death in China of novel reassortant virus. In addition, wild bird migration from Asia to high densities poultry farms population in Java could increase reassortment rate of circulating virus. Furthermore, the finding of A(H3N8) may trigger novel reassortant virus strain with zoonotic potential. Although, human cluster, Tangerang and Karo, is required for further research since the cases occurred only between people with genetic relation.

Acknowledgements

The authors would like to express the highest appreciation to Nugroho, DVM, MSc, (Rosa Farm, Blitar, East Java) for supplying the samples.

Conflict of interest

The authors Khrisdiana Putri, Sitarina Widyarini, Sugiyono and Widya Asmara have no conflict of interest to declare.

Author details

Khrisdiana Putri[1]*, Sitarina Widyarini[2], Sugiyono[2] and Widya Asmara[3]*

1 Department of Veterinary Public Health, Faculty of Veterinary Medicine, Universitas Gadjah Mada, Yogyakarta, Indonesia

2 Department of Pathology, Faculty of Veterinary Medicine, Universitas Gadjah Mada, Yogyakarta, Indonesia

3 Department of Microbiology, Faculty of Veterinary Medicine, Universitas Gadjah Mada, Yogyakarta, Indonesia

*Address all correspondence to: khrisdiana@ugm.ac.id and wied_as@ugm.ac.id

References

[1] Olsen SJ, Ungchusak K, Sovann L, Uyeki TM, Dowell SF, Cox NJ, et al. Family clustering of Avian Influenza A (H5N1). Emerging Infectious Diseases. 2005;**11**(11):1799-1801. Available from: http://www.cdc.gov/eid

[2] Lam T, Hon C-C, Pybus O, Kosakovsky Pond S, Wong R, Yip C-W, et al. Evolutionary and transmission dynamics of reassortant H5N1 influenza virus in Indonesia. PLoS Pathogens. 2008;**4**(8):e1000130

[3] Kandun IN, Wibisono H, Sedyaningsih ER, Yusharmen HW, Purba W, Santoso H, et al. Three Indonesian clusters of H5N1 virus infection in 2005. The New England Journal of Medicine. 2006;**355**(21): 2186-2194. DOI: 10.1056/NEJMoa060930

[4] Setiawaty V, Sedyaningsih ER, Sudiro TM, van Beest Holle MR-DR, Pangesti KN, Ibrahim F. Antibody anti-H5N1 detection in poultry farmers and workers in poultry collection facilities in Indonesia, 2007. Medical Journal of Indonesia. 2010;**19**:124-129

[5] Takano R, Nidom CA, Kiso M, Muramoto Y, Yamada S, Sakai-Tagawa Y, et al. Phylogenetic characterization of H5N1 Avian Influenza Viruses isolated in Indonesia from 2003-2007. Virology. 2009;**390**(1):13-21. DOI: 10.1016/j.virol.2009.04.024

[6] WHO. WHO | Avian Influenza Indonesia—Update 8. World Health Organization. 2011. Available from: http://www.who.int/csr/don/2011_11_15/en/index.html [Accessed: 10 February 2012]

[7] Sedyaningsih ER, Isfandari S, Soendoro T, Supari SF. Towards mutual trust, transparency and equity in virus sharing mechanism: The Avian Influenza case of Indonesia. Annals of the Academy of Medicine, Singapore. 2008;**37**(6):482-488

[8] Dharmayanti NLPI, Thor SW, Zanders N, Hartawan R, Ratnawati A, Jang Y, et al. Attenuation of highly pathogenic Avian Influenza A(H5N1) Viruses in Indonesia following the reassortment and acquisition of genes from low pathogenicity Avian Influenza A Virus progenitors. Emerging Microbes & Infections. 2018;7(1):147. DOI: 10.1038/s41426-018-0147-5

[9] Matrosovich MN, Matrosovich TY, Gray T, Roberts NA, Klenk HD. Human and Avian Influenza Viruses target different cell types in cultures of human airway epithelium. Proceedings of the National Academy of Sciences of the United States of America. 2004;**101**(13):4620-4624. DOI: 10.1073/pnas.0308001101

[10] Thompson CI, Barclay WS, Zambon MC, Pickles RJ. Infection of human airway epithelium by human and avian strains of Influenza A virus. Journal of Virology. 2006;**80**(16):8060-8068. DOI: 10.1128/jvi.00384-06

[11] Vines A, Wells K, Matrosovich M, Castrucci MR, Ito T, Kawaoka Y. The role of influenza A virus hemagglutinin residues 226 and 228 in receptor specificity and host range restriction. Journal of Virology. 1998;**72**(9):7626-7631

[12] Gambaryan A, Tuzikov A, Pazynina G, Bovin N, Balish A, Klimov A. Evolution of the receptor binding phenotype of influenza A (H5) viruses. Virology. 2006;**344**(2):432-438. DOI: 10.1016/j.virol.2005.08.035

[13] Glaser L, Stevens J, Zamarin D, Wilson IA, Garcia-Sastre A, Tumpey TM, et al. A single amino acid substitution in 1918 Influenza virus hemagglutinin changes receptor

binding specificity. Journal of Virology. 2005;**79**(17):11533-11536. DOI: 10.1128/jvi.79.17.11533-11536.2005

[14] Harvey R, Martin AC, Zambon M, Barclay WS. Restrictions to the adaptation of influenza A virus H5 hemagglutinin to the human host. Journal of Virology. 2004;**78**(1):502-507

[15] Shao W, Li X, Goraya MU, Wang S, Chen J-L. Evolution of Influenza A virus by mutation and re-assortment. International Journal of Molecular Sciences. 2017;**18**(8):1650. DOI: 10.3390/ijms18081650

[16] Peiris M, Yen HL. Animal and human influenzas. Revue Scientifique Et Technique (International Office Of Epizootics). 2014;**33**(2):539-553

[17] Stevens J, Blixt O, Tumpey TM, Taubenberger JK, Paulson JC, Wilson IA. Structure and receptor specificity of the hemagglutinin from an H5N1 influenza virus. Science. 2006;**312**(5772):404-410. DOI: 10.1126/science.1124513

[18] Neumann G, Kawaoka Y. Host range restriction and pathogenicity in the context of influenza pandemic. Emerging Infectious Diseases. 2006;**12**(6):881-886

[19] Wibowo MH, Anggoro D, Amanu S, Wahyuni A, Untari T, Artanto S, et al. Receptor binding and antigenic site analysis of hemagglutinin gene fragments of Avian Influenza Virus serotype H5N1 isolated from Indonesia. Pakistan Veterinary Journal. 2017;**2**(37):123-128

[20] OIE. Immediate notification report of Avian Influenza report in Indonesia. 2011. Report reference: Ref OIE:10521 [Report date: 26 April 2011]

[21] Wibawa H, Henning J, Wong F, Selleck P, Junaidi A, Bingham J, et al. A molecular and antigenic survey of H5N1 highly pathogenic Avian Influenza Virus isolates from smallholder duck farms in Central Java, Indonesia during 2007-2008. Virology Journal. 2011;**8**:425-425

[22] Wang SF, Huang JC, Lee YM, Liu SJ, Chan YJ, Chau YP, et al. DC-SIGN mediates avian H5N1 influenza virus infection in Cis and in trans. Biochemical and Biophysical Research Communications. 2008;**373**(4):561-566. DOI: 10.1016/j.bbrc.2008.06.078

[23] Dharmayanti NLPI, Risza Hartawan P, Hendra Wibawa H, Balish A, Donis R, Davis CT, et al. Genetic characterization of clade 2.3.2.1 Avian Influenza A (H5N1) viruses, Indonesia, 2012. Emerging Infectious Diseases. 2014;**20**(4):671-674

[24] Asmara W, Putri K, Tabbu CR. Genetic mapping and study of molecular evolution on Avian Influenza Virus (AIV) H5N1 in Jembrana District, Klungkung District and City of Denpasar, Bali Province, Indonesia: Host radiance analysis. Working Paper. Faculty of Veterinary Medicine, Universitas Gadjah Mada; 2009

[25] Asmara W, Tabbu CR, Wibowo MH. Genetic mapping and study of molecular evolution on Avian Influenza Virus (AIV) H5N1 in Jembrana District, Klungkung District and City of Denpasar, Bali Province, Indonesia: Host radiance analysis. Working Paper. Faculty of Veterinary Medicine, Universitas Gadjah Mada; 2011

[26] Songserm T, Amonsin A, Jam-on R, Sae-Heng N, Meemak N, Pariyothorn N, et al. Avian Influenza H5N1 in naturally infected domestic cat. Emerging Infectious Diseases. 2006;**12**(4):681-683. DOI: 10.3201/eid1204.051396

[27] Nidom CA, Takano R, Yamada S, Sakai-Tagawa Y, Daulay S, Aswadi D, et al. Influenza A (H5N1) viruses from pigs, Indonesia. Emerging Infectious Diseases. 2010;**10**(10):1515-1523

[28] Liu D, Shi W, Gao GF. Poultry carrying H9N2 act as incubators for novel human Avian Influenza Viruses. Lancet. 2014;**383**(9920):869. DOI: 10.1016/s0140-6736(14)60386-x

[29] Azhar M, Lubis A, Siregar E, Alders R, Brum E, McGrane J, et al. Participatory disease surveillance and response in Indonesia: Strengthening veterinary services and empowering communities to prevent and control highly pathogenic Avian Influenza. Avian Diseases. 2010;**54**(1 Suppl):749-753

[30] Siregar ES, Darminto J, Weaver A, Bouma. The vaccination programme in Indonesia. Developments in Biologicals. 2007;**130**:151-158

[31] Swayne D. Principles for vaccine protection in chickens and domestic waterfowl against Avian Influenza: Emphasis on Asian H5N1 high pathogenicity Avian Influenza. Annals of the New York Academy of Sciences. 2006;**1081**:174-181

[32] Swayne DE. Vaccines for List A poultry diseases: Emphasis on Avian Influenza. Developments in Biologicals. 2003;**114**:201-212

[33] Peyre M, Fusheng G, Desvaux S, Roger F. Avian Influenza vaccines: A practical review in relation to their application in the field with a focus on the Asian experience. Epidemiology and Infection. 2009;**137**(1):1-21. DOI: 10.1017/S0950268808001039

[34] Capua I, Terregino C, Cattoli G, Mutinelli F, Rodriguez JF. Development of a DIVA (differentiating infected from vaccinated animals) strategy using a vaccine containing a heterologous neuraminidase for the control of Avian Influenza. Avian Pathology. 2003;**32**(1):47-55. DOI: 10.1080/0307945021000070714

[35] Bouma A, Muljono AT, Jatikusumah A, Nell AJ, Mudjiartiningsih S, Dharmayanti I, et al. Field trial for assessment of Avian Influenza vaccination effectiveness in Indonesia. Revue Scientifique et Technique - Office International des Epizooties. 2008;**27**(3):633-642

[36] Suarez DL. Overview of Avian Influenza DIVA test strategies. Biologicals. 2005;**33**:221-226

[37] Tumpey TM, Alvarez R, Swayne DE, Suarez DL. Diagnostic approach for differentiating infected from vaccinated poultry on the basis of antibodies to NS1, the nonstructural protein of influenza A virus. Journal of Clinical Microbiology. 2005;**43**(2):676-683. DOI: 10.1128/JCM.43.2.676-683.2005

[38] Hadifar F, Ignjatovic J, Tarigan S, Indriani R, Ebrahimie E, Hasan NH, et al. Multimeric recombinant M2e protein-based ELISA: A significant improvement in differentiating Avian Influenza infected chickens from vaccinated ones. PLoS One. 2014;**9**(10):e108420. DOI: 10.1371/journal.pone.0108420

[39] Hemmatzadeh F, Sumarningsih TS, Indriani R, Dharmayanti NL, Ebrahimie E, Ignjatovic J. Recombinant M2e protein-based ELISA: A novel and inexpensive approach for differentiating Avian Influenza infected chickens from vaccinated ones. PLoS One. 2013;**8**(2):e56801. DOI: 10.1371/journal.pone.0056801

[40] Khurana S, Sasono P, Fox A, Nguyen V, Le Q, Pham Q, et al. H5N1-SeroDetect EIA and rapid test: A novel differential diagnostic assay for serodiagnosis of H5N1 infections and surveillance. Journal of Virology. 2011;**85**(23):12455-12463

[41] Putri K, Wawegama N, Ignjatovic J, Noormohammadi AH. Characterisation of the antigenic epitopes in the subunit 2 haemagglutinin of Avian Influenza Virus H5N1. Archives of Virology.

2018;**163**(8):2199-2212. DOI: 10.1007/s00705-018-3896-5

[42] Alexander DJ, Lister SA, Johnson MJ, Randall CJ, Thomas PJ. An outbreak of highly pathogenic Avian Influenza in turkeys in Great Britain in 1991. The Veterinary Record. 1993;**132**(21):535-536

[43] Rebel JM, Peeters B, Fijten H, Post J, Cornelissen J, Vervelde L. Highly pathogenic or low pathogenic Avian Influenza Virus subtype H7N1 infection in chicken lungs: Small differences in general acute responses. Veterinary Research. 2011;**42**:10. DOI: 10.1186/1297-9716-42-10

[44] Pantin-Jackwood MJ, Swayne DE. Pathogenesis and pathobiology of Avian Influenza Virus infection in birds. Revue Scientifique et Technique. 2009;**28**(1):113-136

[45] Mutinelli F, Capua I, Terregino C, Cattoli G. Clinical, gross, and microscopic findings in different avian species naturally infected during the H7N1 low- and high-pathogenicity Avian Influenza epidemics in Italy during 1999 and 2000. Avian Diseases. 2003;**47**(3 Suppl):844-848. DOI: 10.1637/0005-2086-47.s3.844

[46] Acland HM, Silverman Bachin LA, Eckroade RJ. Lesions in broiler and layer chickens in an outbreak of highly pathogenic Avian Influenza Virus infection. Veterinary Pathology. 1984;**21**(6):564-569. DOI: 10.1177/030098588402100603

[47] Swayne DE, Beck JR, Mickle TR. Efficacy of recombinant fowl poxvirus vaccine in protecting chickens against a highly pathogenic Mexican-origin H5N2 Avian Influenza Virus. Avian Diseases. 1997;**41**(4):910-922

[48] Zanella A, Dall'Ara P, Martino PA. Avian Influenza epidemic in Italy due to serovar H7N1. Avian Diseases. 2001;**45**(1):257-261

[49] Soomro SA, Soomro NM, Nizamani ZA, Kalhoro NH, Bughio S. Comparative pathology of experimentally induced Loq pathogenic Avian Influenza (H7N3) infection in chicken, ducks and quails. Pakistan Journal of Agriculture, Agricultural Engineering and Veterinary Sciences. 2016;**32**(2):284-294

[50] de Jong MD, Simmons CP, Thanh TT, Hien VM, Smith GJ, Chau TN, et al. Fatal outcome of human influenza A (H5N1) is associated with high viral load and hypercytokinemia. Nature Medicine. 2006;**12**(10):1203-1207. DOI: 10.1038/nm1477

[51] Ahmed SS, Ersboll AK, Biswas PK, Christensen JP. The space-time clustering of highly pathogenic Avian Influenza (HPAI) H5N1 outbreaks in Bangladesh. Epidemiology and Infection. 2010;**138**(6):843-852. DOI: 10.1017/s0950268810000178

[52] Bertran K, Busquets N, Abad FX, Garcia de la Fuente J, Solanes D, Cordon I, et al. Highly (H5N1) and low (H7N2) pathogenic Avian Influenza Virus infection in Falcons via nasochoanal route and ingestion of experimentally infected prey. PLoS One. 2012;**7**(3):e32107. DOI: 10.1371/journal.pone.0032107

[53] Swayne DE. Selection of and Updating Avian Influenza Vaccine Seed Strains to Maintain Vaccine Efficacy in the Face of Field Virus Drift. 2013. Available from: http://www.offlu.net/fileadmin/home/en/meeting-reports/pdf/OFFLU_Beijing_2013/SWAYNE_D._Process_for_selection_and_evaluation_of_vaccine_seed_strains__and_the_practice_to_update_seed_strains.pdf [Accessed: 24 March 2015]

[54] Wasito R, Wuryastuti H, Pambudy R, Maes RK. Clinical signs and pathologic lesions of highly pathogenic Avian Influenza in Indonesia: A threat to Indonesian poultry. Merit Research

Journal of Microbiology and Biological Sciences. 2016;**4**(1):018-021

[55] Ali A, Elmowalid G, Abdel-Glil M, Sharafeldin T, Abdallah F, Mansour S, et al. Etiology and pathology of epidemic outbreaks of Avian Influenza H5N1 infection in Egyptian chicken farms. Polish Journal of Veterinary Sciences. 2015;**18**(4):779-786. DOI: 10.1515/pjvs-2015-0101

[56] Nili H, Essen S, Nunez A, Banks J, Brown IH. Pathological lesions observed in chickens pre-infected with LP H7N1 A/CK/Italy/1279/99 Avian Influenza and challenged with homologous HP H7N1 A/ostrich/Italy/984/00. Iranian Journal of Veterinary Research. 2008;**9**(3):233-239. DOI: 10.22099/ijvr.2008.570

[57] Elbers AR, Kamps B, Koch G. Performance of gross lesions at postmortem for the detection of outbreaks during the Avian Influenza A Virus (H7N7) epidemic in The Netherlands in 2003. Avian Pathology: Official Journal of the WVPA. 2004;**33**(4):418-422. DOI: 10.1080/03079450410001724030

[58] Damayanti R, Dharmayanti NI, Indriani R, Wiyono A, Darminto. Gambaran Klinis dan Patologis pada Ayam yang Terserang Flu Burung Sangat Patogenik (HPAI) di Beberapa Peternakan di Jawa Timur dan Jawa Barat. JITV. 2004;**9**(2):128-135

[59] Teifke JP, Klopfleisch R, Globig A, Starick E, Hoffmann B, Wolf PU, et al. Pathology of natural infections by H5N1 highly pathogenic Avian Influenza Virus in mute (*Cygnus olor*) and whooper (*Cygnus cygnus*) swans. Veterinary Pathology. 2007;**44**(2):137-143. DOI: 10.1354/vp.44-2-137

[60] Palmai N, Erdelyi K, Balint A, Marton L, Dan A, Deim Z, et al. Pathobiology of highly pathogenic Avian Influenza Virus (H5N1) infection in mute swans (*Cygnus olor*). Avian Pathology: Official Journal of the WVPA. 2007;**36**(3):245-249. DOI: 10.1080/03079450701341957

[61] Wibowo MH, Susetya H, Untari T, Putri K, Tabbu CR, Asmara W. Molecular study on the pathogenicity of Avian Influenza Virus. Indonesian Journal of Biotechnology. 2006;**11**(2):901-907

[62] Swayne DE, Suarez DL, Sims LD. Influenza. In: Swayne DE, Glisson JR, McDougald LR, Nolan LK, Suarez DL, Nair VL, editors. Diseases of Poultry. 13th ed. UK: John Wiley & Sons, Inc; 2013. pp. 181-218. DOI: 10.1002/9781119421481

[63] Kim HR, Kwon YK, Jang I, Lee YJ, Kang HM, Lee EK, et al. Pathologic changes in wild birds infected with highly pathogenic Avian Influenza A(H5N8) Viruses, South Korea, 2014. Emerging Infectious Diseases. 2015;**21**(5):775-780. DOI: 10.3201/eid2105.141967

[64] Swayne DE, Suarez DL. Highly pathogenic Avian Influenza. Revue Scientifique et Technique - Office International des Épizooties. 2000;**19**(2):463-482

[65] Alexander DJ. Current situation of Avian Influenza in poultry in Great Britain Avian Diseases, Vol. 47 (Special Issue—2003). In: First International Symposium on Avian Influenza, 1981 Proceedings; 1982. pp. 35-45

[66] Kobayashi Y, Horimoto T, Kawaoka Y, Alexander DJ, Itakura C. Pathological studies of chickens experimentally infected with two highly pathogenic Avian Influenza viruses. Avian Pathology: Official Journal of the WVPA. 1996;**25**(2):285-304. DOI: 10.1080/03079459608419142

[67] Ellis TM, Bousfield RB, Bissett LA, Dyrting KC, Luk GS, Tsim ST, et al. Investigation of outbreaks of highly

pathogenic H5N1 Avian Influenza in waterfowl and wild birds in Hong Kong in late 2002. Avian Pathology: Official Journal of the WVPA. 2004;**33**(5): 492-505. DOI: 10.1080/03079450400 003601

[68] Brojer C, Agren EO, Uhlhorn H, Bernodt K, Morner T, Jansson DS, et al. Pathology of natural highly pathogenic Avian Influenza H5N1 infection in wild tufted ducks (*Aythya fuligula*). Journal of Veterinary Diagnostic Investigation: Official Publication of the American Association of Veterinary Laboratory Diagnosticians, Inc. 2009;**21**(5):579-587. DOI: 10.1177/104063870902100501

[69] Chaves AJ, Busquets N, Campos N, Ramis A, Dolz R, Rivas R, et al. Pathogenesis of highly pathogenic Avian Influenza A virus (H7N1) infection in chickens inoculated with three different doses. Avian Pathology: Official Journal of the WVPA. 2011;**40**(2):163-172. DOI: 10.1080/03079457.2011.551874

[70] Klopfleisch R, Wolf PU, Wolf C, Harder T, Starick E, Niebuhr M, et al. Encephalitis in a Stone Marten (*Martes foina*) after natural infection with highly pathogenic Avian Influenza Virus subtype H5N1. Journal of Comparative Pathology. 2007;**137**(2):155-159. DOI: 10.1016/j.jcpa.2007.06.001

Chapter 7

Adequate Monitor of Avian Influenza Viral Infections and Foresight About Possibilities of Its Human Epidemic and Pandemic Infections

Yuji Takemoto

Abstract

Avian influenza viruses are shared among wild birds and sometimes are shed from wild birds to domestic poultry and backyard domestic animals. Usually avian influenza viruses infect wild birds as asymptomatic or low pathogenesis and are stocked in birds, water, and soil. Accumulation of genetic changes of influenza viruses in hosts diversities the pathogenesis to hosts described as highly pathogenic avian influenza viruses and low pathogenic avian influenza viruses. Highly pathogenic avian influenza viruses being categorized among influenza A subtype viruses (H5, H7, H9) and different from low pathogenic avian influenza viruses cause severe illness and sudden increased deaths of wild birds, chicken, or other poultry. These infect from avian to humans. The adequate approaches of information and action for appearance of HPAI and LPAI viral infections in flock may prohibit the outbreak of avian to humans, which are mostly including quarantine of the infected area of the flock from surrounding laboratory tests for HPAI and LPAI viruses in early illness and antiviral treatments in humans.

Keywords: zoonotic infection, antigenic drift, antigenic shift, influenza A virus strain

1. Introduction

There are four types of influenza viruses, types A, B, C, and D, in the world. Influenza virus infection is zoonotic and sometimes restricted to specific species. Influenza A and B viruses mainly cause disease among humans, swine, and avian. Influenza C virus infects humans and swine but does not cause severe disease, and its infection to humans is rarely reported [1]. Influenza D viruses affect swine and cattle and are not known to cause sickness to humans [1]. Influenza B viruses infect humans and avian and cause epidemic in the limiting mild disease [2]. Influenza B virus is concerned about seasonal viral infection but not endemic or pandemic. Influenza A virus is different from other types of influenza viruses about the wide infectious ranges of host and severity of disease. Influenza A viruses are theoretically classified into thousands of different antigenic subtypes by the combinations of the main viral antigens: hemagglutinin (HA) and neuraminidase (NA) [3]. Recently 18 different HA subtypes and 11 different NA subtypes have been identified [4, 5]. Influenza A viruses are classified from H1N1 to H18N11 and are called as avian influenza virus, swine influenza virus, or other types of animal influenza viruses depending on original infectious host. Humans, swine, and avian are infective host of influenza A virus, but infectious influenza A viral subtypes among intraspecies are restricted by the binding affinity of the HA protein to sialyloligosaccharides (oligosaccharides containing terminal silica acids linked to galactose) on host cell surface glycoprotein or glycolipids [6]. Influenza A viruses cause normally self-limited disease (asymptomatic or mild) and are shared with humans and many different animals. Most subtypes of influenza A viruses are primarily reserved in aquatic birds, are distinct from human influenza A viruses, and do not easily transmit to human due to host species barriers [7]. Zoonotic infection between humans and animals or interspecies of infection of influenza A viruses makes viral evolutions which can help to surmount species barriers [8]. Avian influenza viruses transmit from aquatic birds to poultry and change virus properties and result in change pathogenesis ranging from mild disease to severe disease with high death rates in host species. According to these phenomena, avian influenza viruses cause severe disease and high death rate in host, which are called as highly pathogenic avian influenza (HPAI) viruses, and avian influenza viruses result in mild disease or asymptomatic infection to host, which are called as low pathogenic avian influenza (LPAI) viruses. A virus is defined as HPAI or LPAI by its ability to cause disease and mortality in intravenously inoculated young chickens in the laboratory or by its possession of molecular characteristic features associated with HPAI viruses. Avian, swine, and other zoonotic influenza infections in humans may happen on the condition of the successful transmission with the sufficient contact between donor and recipient species, successful species jumps of influenza viruses, the influenza viral complex adaptations, and achieved sustained transmission in a new species [7]. Those may cause several ranges of disease in humans depending on viral factors and human factors [9]. HPAI virus infections have been monitored from avian to humans and caused the endemic disease of high fatality rate [10]. HPAI viruses may cause pandemic from endemic on the condition of no effective protection for wide shedding of HPAI viruses. Monitoring of disease severity of avian and human influenza A virus infection could prevent the severe damage to the society from the emerging infectious disease of influenza A viruses [9].

2. Evolution of influenza A viruses

2.1 Antigenic drift

Influenza viruses cause annual recurrent epidemics in humans, which approximately result in 3–5 million cases of severe illness and 250,000–500,000 deaths worldwide [11]. Most of these were occurred by influenza A and B viruses. Especially influenza A viruses change viral surface glycoproteins HA and NA by accumulations of point mutations in HA and NA genes and escape from human immunity called as antigenic drift, which may occur as seasonal influenza epidemic. But antigenic drift does not evolve virulence of influenza A viruses which cause severe disease in humans [12]. Seasonal influenza viral infections are limiting disease and mild, which cause severe disease and death by factors of host immune conditions. This does not mean that there is no necessity of treatment of anti-influenza viral therapy for seasonal influenza infections. The adequate diagnosis and treatment for seasonal influenza infection diminish severe illness and subsequent death from seasonal influenza infections and lead to awareness of emerging infectious disease [13].

2.2 Avian influenza A H5N1 viruses

In 1997 HPAI (H5N1) viruses occurred among wild birds and caused an outbreak in poultry and sporadic human infection in Hong Kong [14]. This was firstly identified as the crossover of avian-human species barrier and resulted in 18 infected individuals and 6 of 18 patients died [15]. Zoonotic infection of avian influenza virus H5N1 has been widely spread from Asia to Europe and Africa, which has been endemic in some countries and caused outbreaks resulting in millions of poultry infections, several hundreds of human infectious cases, and many human deaths since 2003 [16]. Avian influenza virus H5N1 causes a disease which has aggressive symptoms different from a mild disease of seasonal influenza virus infection in humans [9]. HA is a surface viral protein which binds to and uses sialic acid-containing molecules as receptors for viral infection to multiple cells. Avian influenza virus strains circulated in waterfowl contain HAs with preference for binding to sialic acids linked to the rest of the sugar by an α2–3 linkage. In contrast, HAs from human influenza virus strains show enhanced binding to α2–6-linked sialic acids [17]. Seasonal influenza viruses cause symptoms of upper respiratory infection by correlation with an abundance of α2–6-linked sialic acids in the upper respiratory tract of humans [18]. More detailed analysis of H5N1 infection showed an abundance of α2–3-linked sialic acids in the lower respiratory tract of humans, and the explanation of severe disease of the lung was done, as pneumonia and respiratory failure in H5N1 infection [19]. In addition to an abundance of avian influenza viral receptor in lower respiratory tract in humans, the autopsy reports of H5N1-infected patients revealed avian influenza virus infection intra and extra lung concluding the brain, intestine, heart, spleen, lymphoid tissue, kidney, and placenta by applying immunohistochemistry (IHC) with monoclonal antibodies to hemagglutinin (HA) and nucleocapsid protein (NP) and/or in situ hybridization with sense and antisense probes to HA and NP to detect viral antigens and genomic sequences in various organs of H5N1 cases and RT-PCR and nucleic acid sequence-based amplification H5 detection assays [20–25]. HAs with multiple residues at the cleavage site of precursor HAs that can be activated by ubiquitous intracellular proteases may cause systemic infections; on the other hand, HAs with a single arginine residue at the cleavage site of precursor HAs that can only be cleaved by extracellular trypsin-like proteases present in the upper respiratory and gastrointestinal tracts may give rise to local infections [26]. The disease severity in human cases varies from mild to extremely severe; mutations of HA may always be related to the ability of receptor binding but not the virulence of viruses, which imply that there are other factors responsible for the virulence of H5N1 influenza viruses in humans [27]. As the characterization of avian influenza A H5N1, the analysis of H5N1 infections showed the deletion of 19 amino acids of the stalk region in NA protein that cleaves and separates the HA of progeny virions from the sialic acid-containing receptors on the surface of the infected host cells, in which they were generated [14, 28]. This deletion may play a role in the transmission of virus across species [29]. The polymerase complex is composed of three viral polymerase proteins
(PB1, PB2, and PA) involved in viral RNA synthesis. In the polymerase complex of avian influenza viruses, glutamic acid to lysine substitution at position 627 of PB2 was isolated but not a prerequisite for high virulence in humans [30]. The 1918 pandemic was called as Spanish flu and proposed that the 1918 virus was not a reassorted virus (like those of the 1957 and 1968 pandemics), but more likely an entirely

avian-like virus that has adapted to humans. But the 1918 influenza virus was analyzed as 10 amino acids change the polymerase complex including the lysine residue at position 627 [31]. These mutations require more investigation for the precursors of a new influenza pandemic. PB1-F2 is a small mitochondrial protein that is encoded on an open reading frame of PB1 [32]. This open reading frame is highly conserved in avian influenza isolates [33]. The reconstructed 1918 influenza virus linked to the PB1-F2 protein and recombinant virus with a single mutation in the PB1-F2 protein [serine (S) instead of asparagine (N) at position 66] of H5N1 (Hk/97) increase viral pathogenicity [34, 35]. PB1-F2 may induce apoptosis of immune cells and an insufficient adaptive immune response [35]. The NS proteins (NS1 and NS2) are viral proteins, and NS1 has multiple functions including splicing and nuclear export of cellular mRNA as well as stimulation of translation [36]. The NS1 protein is crucial for evading the innate immune response of the host by inhibiting the antiviral response mediated by type I interferons [37]. The presence of glutamic acid at position 92 of NS1 has been investigated to be a prerequisite for the resistance to antiviral cytokines considering the results of severe disease induction by inoculation of reassortant influenza virus (H1N1) bearing the NS gene of the H5N1/97 virus to pigs and the lack of glutamic acid at position of the NS1 protein in the recent human and avian isolates [38–41]. Two PDZ ligand (PL) sequence motifs (a Glu-Pro-Glu-Val (EPEV), a Glu-Ser-Glu-Val (ESEV)) were detected in viruses isolated during 1997 but not in viruses after 1997 as a potential codominants of virulence disrupting several PDZ-domain protein-mediated pathways for cell signaling [33].

M1 and M2 are matrix proteins, and M2 is a 97-residue single-pass membrane protein with its N-terminus directed toward the outside of the virus. It determines proton selectivity and unidirectional conductance of the channel by mutagenesis studies [42]. A serine to asparagine substitution at residue 31 of M2 protein is associated with resistance to adamantanes which were used for therapy of influenza A virus infections [43]. On the other hand, M2 protein is suggested to be a candidate for the adaptation of the virus to a new host in addition to PB1-F2 from a study of Thai and Indonesian isolates [43].

2.3 Avian influenza A H7N9 viruses

Avian influenza viruses sometimes infect poultry as LPAI, and there is no concern to LPAI, but even LPAI suddenly caused the sporadic infection among humans which started on February 19, 2013, in Shanghai [44]. There was no epidemic of severe disease in poultry infections with H7N9 before human infections with H7N9. In April 2013, the number of human cases of H7N9 virus infections increased significantly, reaching 125 confirmed cases in China, which was suggested to be derived from contacting with poultry and/or contaminated environments in farmers' markets with live birds [45]. After closure of live birds' markets, the number of new human cases infected with H7N9 declined rapidly. But the second wave of human infections with H7N9 virus started again owing to the lower fall temperature and reopening of poultry markets in the fall of 2013. This wave is characterized by the extensive geographic spread from the province of Eastern China to Southern China and a large number of human infections with H7N9 (440 human infections and 122 associated death of 440 as of May 16, 2014) [46]. For the protection of widespread of H7H9, two strategies composed of suspending farmers' markets with live birds and stopping the transport for trading of live birds carrying the virus were applied by provincial and Chinese authorities [47, 48]. These measures controlled the more spread of H7N9 virus infections in China, but the potential benefits of public health measures should be balanced against the potentially significant societal and economic costs [49]. The lack of protective antibodies in human against

H7N9 virus leads to the result of influenza pandemic in humans, nevertheless of zoonotic infection of poultry to humans [50]. During October 1, 2016–August 7, 2017, the largest fifth epidemic of Asian H7N9 infections since 2013 was reported as 759 human infections including 281 deaths [51]. The total of human infections has reached to 1557 human infections and at least 605 deaths (39%) during March 31, 2013–August 7, 2017 [51]. Fourteen clusters of two or three persons with H7N9 happened during the fifth epidemic Asian H7N9 that was explained in association with wider geographic spread and higher prevalence of Asian virus among poultry and not as a result of any increased incidence of poultry to humans or human-to-human spread [51]. In the genesis of H7N9, H7 of H7N9 is derived from H7N3 viruses isolated among ducks in Eastern China in 2010–2011, and N9 of H7N9 is derived from avian H2N9 and/or H11N9 viruses isolated among wild migratory birds along the East Asian flyway [50, 52]. Both of them are Eurasian lineage of avian viruses, and reassortment of gene (so-called as antigenic shift) may happen and produce the possible precursor of H7N9 virus. Six viral genes except H7 and N9 of H7N9 virus likely originated from chicken H9N2 sub-lineages 1 and 2 circulating in Eastern China [50, 52]. Antigenic shift is suggested to form H7N9 virus during the generation and evolution of viruses. In the analysis of H7N9, viral sequences revealed that H7N9 virus possesses leucine or isoleucine at position 226 of HA which binds to both sialic acid-α2,3-galactose (avian-type receptor) and sialic acid-α2,6-galactose (human -type receptor) [53]. This may mean as the avian virus infection to humans in addition to expression of sialic acid-α2,6-galactose in the upper respiratory tract and sialic acid-α2,3-galactose in the lower respiratory tract in humans [19, 21–25]. According to PB2 protein of H7N9, sequence analysis revealed that many isolated H7N9 viruses encode lysine at position 627 of PB2 [54]. This substitution of glutamic acid (E) to lysine (K) of position 627 of PB2 (E627K mutation) may enable avian viruses to adapt to efficient replication at 33 and 37°C of human temperature lower than original avian host temperature (41°C) [55, 56]. Other mutations of position 627 of PB2 in these viruses have been reported and investigated [56]. The resistant H7N9 variants encoding the R294K mutation in NA that confers resistance to oseltamivir have been detected in patients treated with neuraminidase inhibitors (NAIs). R294K substitution was revealed as multidrug resistance with extreme oseltamivir resistance by the study of using protein- and virus-based assays [57]. On the other hand, K294 mutation of H7N9 infections was found. Compared with H7N9 viruses containing K294 which leads to mild resistance to NAIs, R294K appeared in clinical course under the selective pressure of oseltamivir treatment and conferred not only multidrug resistance to NAIs but also decreases NA activity and impaired virus replication. These phenomena may explain the failure for predominance of R294K-mutated strains of H7N9 in this outbreak. But the drug-resistant mutations should be monitored vigilantly in order to help the most effective drug administration and the prevention of unnecessary loss of human lives in clinical course [57]. Recently LPAI H7N9 viruses have evolved to HPAI viruses and caused the increased morbidity and mortality in poultry, and the same phenomenon has more likely occurred in human infections [51].

2.4 Avian influenza A H7N7 viruses

Outbreaks of HPAI virus infections mostly originate from endemic LPAI viral strains of H5 and H7 subtypes among wild waterfowl. These LPAI virus strains can transmit from waterfowl to poultry and change virulence to HPA virus among poultry [58]. In the Netherlands, an epidemic of HPAI virus H7N7 infection occurred in 2003 that resulted in 255 affected flocks and culling (killing and removing of infected poultry flocks) of 30 million birds [59]. Control measures were applied to HPAI virus infection in poultry leading to the potential start of human influenza pandemic, such as culling and banning the movement of infected flocks and tracing and screening of the infection which were implemented, followed by preemptive culling of flocks in a 1-km zone around the infected flock. In this HPAI viral epidemic in poultry, 86 poultry workers and 3 household contacts were identified to be affected with H7N7 by RT-PCR, and the main symptom of this infection was conjunctivitis (83/89 persons) and one fatal case happened [60, 61]. Since 2006–2011 LPAI virus infection in the Netherlands (2006) and in Germany (2011) and HPAI virus infection in England (2008) and in Spain (2009), H7N7 viral infections were reported. These show the difficulty in the elimination of epidemic avian influenza viral infection from the endemic avian influenza virus infection among wild waterfowls. As additional measures, vaccination for poultry in outbreaks of H7N7 significantly reduced the excretion of viruses, which may reduce virus spread in infected areas and the risk of human exposure to viruses, in Italy (2000) [62]. Compared with the H7N1 and H7N3 episodes leading no bird to human transmission in Italy, in the genetic analysis of H7N7, HA gene of H7N7 is quite similar to HA genes of H7N1 and H7N3. So other mutations in NA or internal genes of H7N7 virus including E627K in PB2 except HA may determine the capacity to replicate and cause disease in humans. Although H7N7 virus may replicate well in the human cells near the eyes, it may not well replicate in the human upper respiratory tract [61].

2.5 Avian influenza A H9N2 viruses

Influenza virus A H9N2 has been firstly known in 1966 as the infection among turkeys in Wisconsin. Until 1998–1999, influenza H9N2 viruses are less considered to be as zoonotic transmission, although this H9N2 widespread is nearly global including several Asian countries among from wild birds to domestic poultry populations [63]. H9N2 viruses are characterized as LPAI viruses that have caused mild disease which led to decreased egg production and deaths in poultry [64]. In China, natural human infections with H9N2 were firstly reported as seropositive cases in Guangdong province in 1998 and several cases with mild or asymptomatic illness in the South or mainland China and Hong Kong in 1999 [65]. H9N2 LPAI viruses, that were isolated from an infected human in Pakistan in 2012–2015 and in Northern China in 2017, have an identical amino acid residue leucine at 226 in the receptor binding site of HA, the C-terminus of PDZ ligand motif in NS1 (KSEI), NP (E372D), and L55F in the M2 protein that are mammalian host-specific markers [64, 66]. Avian influenza H9N2 viral infections have been globally distributed as mild and asymptomatic infection in humans, poultry, pet birds, and other domestic animals and may trigger weak immune responses and production of low titer of antibody to H9N2 in humans [63, 66]. These were inducted as infections from poultry to humans directly or indirectly, but not as human-to-human transmission [63, 66]. Low rates of influenza A H9N2 viral infection in poultry-exposed individuals may cause an epidemic with a longer duration or a greater magnitude than if the virus was introduced to a completely unexposed population [67]. H9N2 also demonstrates its potential to efficient transmission from avian hosts and sharing genetic materials (e.g., internal genes) with other viruses as appearance of H7N9 and H10N8 [68, 69].

2.6 Other avian viruses in human infections: H10N8, H5N6, H7N2, H7N3, H6N1, and H10N7

In China in 2013, human infection of avian influenza A H10N8 virus was firstly reported as severe illness which resulted in death within 9 days of clinical course [69].

This strain is different from others isolated from poultry and wild birds and reassortant of H9N2 containing genetic markers for mammalian adaptation and virulence in HA (A135T, S138A), M1 (N30D, T215A), NS1 (P42S), and PB2 (E627K). This virus was sensitive to neuraminidase inhibitors (NAIs) [69].

In China in 2014, human infection of avian influenza virus was caused by H5N6 HPAI virus following the epidemic infections of many birds' death [70]. Until 2017, a total of 16 human cases infected with avian influenza H5N6 and 11 fatal cases of 16 cases (an overall CFR of 69%) were reported [71]. Thirteen of 16 cases had exposure to live poultry or live poultry markets (LPMs). Avian influenza H5N6 viruses belonged to HA H5 genetic clade 2.3.4.4 have evolved from H5N1 and H9N2 viruses [72], and similar H5 clade A (H5N6) viruses have been detected in wild birds and poultry in China, Japan, Lao People's Democratic Republic, Myanmar, the Republic of Korea, and Vietnam [73]. Analyses of poultry and environmental samples indicate that the different avian influenza A H5N6 virus genotypes may vary by geographic regions as HPAI viruses or LPAI viruses [73].

In the United States of America (USA) in 2016, avian influenza A H7N2 infected one human after an outbreak of infection among cats in an animal shelter in New York City. This person's infection was associated with close contact with sick cats affected with H7N2-isolated virus and no widespread to any other persons [74]. Avian influenza H7N2 viral infection to humans has been reported as the result of prolonged long contact with infected birds since 2002 in the USA. But the screening of more than 350 people with exposure to infected cats during this outbreak appeared no more human infection except one, and the risk posed by this virus to the public was thought to be low. Isolated H7N2 viruses in the USA are characterized as LPAI virus but have increased binding to sialic acid-α2,6-galactose receptor and reduced binding to sialic acid-α2,3-galactose receptor which has the possibility of human-to-human infection [75].

In Canada in 2004, a two-time outbreak of avian influenza A H7N3 viral infection happened in one farm: the first was characterized as LPAI viral infection which resulted in 8–16 deaths/day among 9200 chickens in a barn, and the second was detected as HPAI viral infection which resulted in 2000 deaths in 2 days among 9030 chickens in an adjacent barn [76]. After the outbreaks of LPAI and HPAI virus infections, the examination of testing for H7N3 among approximately 2000 poultry farm workers and 650 workers assisted with outbreak management and control revealed 57 suspected and/or confirmed as avian influenza infections [76]. Only two confirmed patients with avian influenza A H7N3 virus had conjunctivitis and mild influenza-like illness cases infected with avian influenza A H7N7 virus in the Netherlands.

In Taiwan in 2013, a human infection with avian influenza A H6N1 was recognized as mild pneumonia and quick improvement by treated oseltamivir. A 20-year-old woman works at a breakfast shop and had not been exposed to poultry or birds and no travel to China. Investigation of 36 close contacts with her cleared no positive tests for avian influenza A H6N1, and two poultry farms within 1 km from the woman's house were investigated as the results of no H6N1 virus infection [77]. Avian influenza A H6N1 virus strain commonly circulates in domestic birds in Taiwan, and this infection happened to be found in the alert of a Taiwanese traveler's infection with epidemic avian influenza H7N9 virus in China in 2013. Genetic and structural analysis of isolated H6N1 virus reveals that a single nucleotide substitution resulting in a change from Gly to Asp at position 225 of HA (G225D) leads to direct interaction of Asp225 with the penultimate of Gal of the human-type receptor and the stabilized binding to human receptor [78]. E627K mutation in PB2 is well known to human adaptation of avian influenza viruses but is not present in avian and human isolates.

In Australia in 2010, an outbreak of LPAI H10N7 viruses was identified as 10–25 bird's deaths for 8–14 days, a 15% decrease of egg production, and no respiratory signs in affected flocks. Two of seven abattoirs who had conjunctivitis and minor upper respiratory tract symptoms were identified to be infected by H10N7 virus [79]. In Australia in 2010, surveillance for H10N7 viruses showed small numbers of wild waterfowl on the affected site and no infection of H10 subtypes in poultry around 2 km of affected farms.

2.7 Other strains of avian influenza viruses.

In addition to avian influenza strains of poultry to human infections, epidemics of avian influenza A strains are reported: H5N2, H5N5, and H5N8 viruses as HPAI viruses and H3N8, H6N6, H10N4, H10N5, H11N2, and H7N8 as occasional infection to mammals.

3. Transmission of species

3.1 Genes' transport of wild birds to poultry by antigenic shift

As above, many avian influenza reasssortant viruses have emerged during viral transmission from wild birds (donor spices) to poultry (recipient species). LPAI viruses from wild birds have been reasserted with other influenza virus strains of poultry and changed virulence in poultry. If LPAI viruses could not adapt to new host of poultry, they would die out. LPAI viruses have been environmentally sustained by close contact to LPAI viruses among wild birds when avian influenza A virus infections happened in endemic countries. Host species barriers do not mean simply the biological barriers [7]. Biological barriers between wild birds and poultry are almost the same in concerning about influenza binding receptor in cell membrane (α2–3-linked sialic acids) and replication condition in host temperature [19, 53]. In addition to biological barriers, interspecific interactions between wild birds (donor) and poultry (recipient), interactions between avian influenza viruses and poultry (recipient), and interactions among individuals of poultry (recipient) are considered as environmental barriers [7]. In consequence of surmounting these barriers, LPAI viruses have been sustained by the successful onward adaptation to new hosts like H7N7 viruses, H9N2 viruses and H7N9 viruses in the present [47, 59, 64]. If humans have been in close contact to poultry affected with LPAI viruses, asymptomatic or mild illness of avian influenza A virus infections would appear in humans but rarely leads to fatal disease [45, 46]. LPAI viruses suddenly have changed virulence to HPAI viruses and caused severe disease and deaths among poultry like the emergence of H5N1 virus being in consequent to human epidemic [14]. Increased virulence from LPAI to HPAI following antigenic shift could not be predicted before the happening. Avian influenza A viruses need to acquire the abilities to transmit to new host species and replicate effectively in new host before an epidemic or pandemic [7]. Antigenic shift in avian viruses has transmitted the abilities of transferring from poultry to humans and replicating progeny in humans by accumulated mutations in HA, NA, PB2, NS1, etc. but has not transmitted the abilities of transferring from human to human [28–38].

3.2 Possibility of intermediate hosts or mixing vessels for the generation for pandemic influenza viruses

Avian has α2–3-linked sialic acids, human has α2–6-linked sialic acids, and swine has both types of receptor for HA of influenza A viruses [80]. These enable

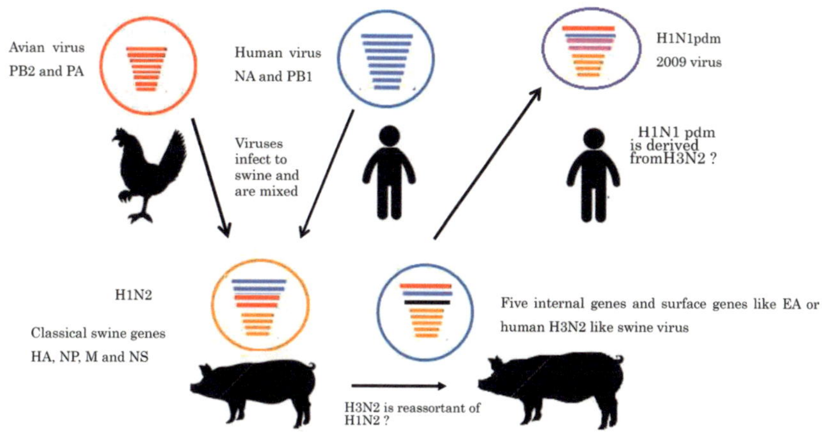

Figure 1.
Reassortant H1N2 influenza viruses and H1N1 pdm 2009 in swine.

pigs to be susceptible to both human and avian influenza viruses. If a human influenza A virus infection and an avian influenza A virus infection happened simultaneously in swine, antigenic shift may produce new pandemic viruses which can be transmitted easily from person to person among human population with little or no immune response to them. In China, avian-like H1N1 and novel reassortant H1N2 influenza viruses from pigs were reported [81]. The swine H1N1 virus (A/swine/Zhejiang/1/07) was close to avian-like H1N1 viruses which is seemed to be derived from the European swine H1N1 viruses, and the two H1N2 viruses (A/swine/Shanghai/1/07 and A/swine/Guangxi/13/06) were novel reassortant H1N2 influenza viruses containing genes from the classical swine (HA, NP, M, and NS), human (NA and PB1), and avian (PB2 and PA) lineage, which indicated that the reassortment of influenza viruses happened among humans, avian, and swine and the generation of new viruses was produced in swine [81]. In the analysis of influenza virus H1N1 pdm in 2009, the main persistent pdm/09-origin reassortant forms had at least five pdm/09-origin internal genes, and their surface genes were primarily of European avian-like (EA) or human H3N2-like swine influenza virus [82] (**Figure 1**). The monitor for a new pandemic virus is necessary to monitor and survey the epidemic infection in swine, in addition to monitoring of endemic LPAI infections among wild birds and poultry, epidemic LPAI and HPAI infections among wilds birds and poultry, and the following human infections by LPAI and HPAI viruses.

4. Systemic monitor and approach for a new information of epidemic and pandemic infections

Avian influenza viral infections are wide ranges of mammalians, and it is not enough to monitor avian, swine, and humans for covering all types of avian influenza virus infection because of the rare case appearance of the LPAI outbreak in cats in the USA [74]. The World Health Organization (WHO) continuously monitors avian and other zoonotic influenza viruses closely through its Global Influenza Surveillance and Response System (GISRS) (http://www.who.int/influenza/gisrslaboratory/en/). From this site, necessary information about occurrence of outbreaks, conditions, widespread of infections, etc. can be investigated and gathered. But insufficient monitor for zoonotic influenza infections as potential to the human pandemic is reinforced by the information from the collaboration with the World Organization for Animal Health (OIE) (www.oie,int/) and the Food and Agriculture Organization (FAO) (www.fao.org/home/en/). In each country, the national disease center monitors its own country and internationally collaborates with the WHO. Monitoring reinforces the environmental barriers by noticing abnormal wild birds' deaths in a province to the provincial and national authorities in an early stage of an endemic. Following this information, provincial authorities would start to investigate etiology of birds' deaths and any other birds' deaths around this area and water pollution by avian influenza viruses in ponds if avian influenza viruses caused birds' deaths. Environmental barriers have three steps which are composed of a first step of transmission from waterfowl to poultry, a second step of transmission of individuals among poultry, and a third step of transmission from poultry to humans (**Figure 2**). When a first step of environmental barrier from wild birds to poultry is surmounted by avian influenza viruses, two patterns of damage in poultry (asymptomatic/mild disease or severe disease/deaths) are recognized. It is very difficult to detect early and diagnose asymptomatic infections in poultry, but any changes in poultry including coughing and decrease numbers of egg production should not be missed. Recently rapid influenza diagnostic tests (RIDTs) are available in testing for avian influenza viruses (H5, H7, and H9), but other RIDTs for detection of more HA subtypes are desirable to be developed in demand [83]. If any doubt for avian influenza infection, RIDTs are recommended to be applied immediately within the limits of lower sensitivity than RT-PCR and other methods. A combination of RIDTs (infection of avian influenza viruses), RT-PCR (viral genes sequence and subtypes), HA inhibition test (viral subtype), ELISA (all subtypes of avian influenza viruses and widespread of viral infection), and the inoculation of isolated viruses to chicken (identification of viral pathogeny) would be adapted without any time consumption for diagnosis. These tests may provide an initial measure and further measures for control of an endemic, epidemic, and a potential pandemic infection of avian viruses. A second step of environmental barrier is reinforced by using the following measures: isolation of birds from the others, the use of personal protection equipment (PPEs)

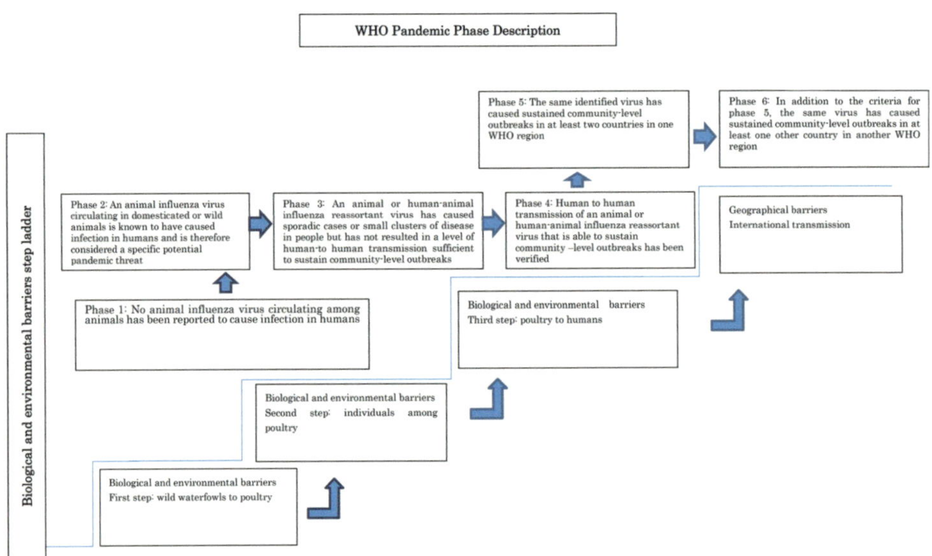

Figure 2.
Comparison WHO Pandemic Phase and biological and environmental barriers step ladder.

by farm workers, and culling the affected birds. But widespread of avian viral infections among poultry is not necessary for a long time. So it is desirable to diagnose avian viral infection in the shortest time since the first notification of disease by these diagnostic tests. Vaccination of poultry has been applied for the prevention from economic damage of culling and a potential pandemic, as biological barriers [84]. But vaccines of animals for avian viral infections would be desired to high efficacy and prevalence use in the areas. Considering the negative effect for the difficulty of conducting surveillance for persistence of the virus after vaccination or insufficient immune response in birds leading to the latent viral infection in poultry, vaccination should carefully be adapted as one component of control measures [84]. Control strategies and measures including technical guidelines for pandemic potential are available from FAO and OIE [84, 85]. It is emphasized that the surveillance standards and methodology are necessary for calling rapid response for containment or mitigation of emerging infectious disease of avian influenza but not a system for rapid detection of emerging novel influenza strains or outbreaks of disease [85]. Sentinel surveillance is desired to protect poultry and humans from the threat of epidemic and/or pandemic potential in the prevalence of avian viruses among wild birds and poultry. Collapse of a third step of environmental barrier is recognized as human infection with avian influenza viruses. This condition is called as pandemic phase 2 in the WHO pandemic phase descriptions [86] (**Figure 2**). Human infection primarily may appear in direct or indirect exposure to infected live or dead poultry or contaminated environments, such as live bird markets. And human infection also may appear concerning slaughtering, de-feathering, handling carcasses of infected poultry, and preparing poultry for consumption, especially in household settings [87]. Surveillance of avian viral infections in these persons will be done by applying combinations of diagnostic methods as soon as possible from the onset of the first poultry infections. Consumption of prepared poultry and raw egg dishes has been reported to be linked with the infection of H5N1 human cases [87]. The virus is inactivated at temperatures (at least 70°C the center of the product) in conventional cooking, and consumption of properly cooked poultry and eggs should be recommended [88]. Although human-to-human transmission of avian influenza viruses may occur in the close and/or prolonged contact with the patients, there has been no sustained human-to-human transmission of these viruses identified [89]. But in North America in 2009, influenza A (H1N1) pdm 009 virus originated from swine influenza viruses surmounted biological barriers. It took only a few months to amount to a total number of 73 affected countries and more than 26,000 laboratory-confirmed infected cases from the first case in Mexico in February of 2009 which is called as pandemic phase 6 (**Figure 2**) [90]. These suggested how fast infections had been spread in the world and how difficult to control the widespread of emerging infectious disease (EID) after the new emerging avian influenza virus had obtained the capacity of the interhuman transmission. In this phase, therapy for patients and adaptation of control measures for pandemic were necessary. Antiviral drugs for influenza viral infections except adamantanes are effective for avian influenza infections in the early stage of infection for the decrease of mortality rate [91]. Administration of neuraminidase inhibitors (NAIs) to infected persons within 48 hours of onset would be recommended, and isolation of infected people from the public would be important in a limited term. Recently baloxavir marboxil that prevents replication by inhibiting the cap-dependent endonuclease activity of the viral polymerase and is effective for seasonal influenza and avian influenza virus infections is available in Japan [92]. In addition to NAIs, it may be one of the powerful tools as antiviral therapy. In the pre-pandemic stage to the pandemic stage, network information and control measures from the national disease center, the Global Influenza Surveillance Network (GISN), Global Outbreak and Alert Network (GOARN), and the original network for influenza viral infection in province. In usual diagnosis and treatment of influenza viral infection, RIDTs are a useful step-up strategy for the treatment of influenza viral infections regardless of limiting sensitivity. RIDTs for seasonal influenza viral infection can only detect A type and/or B type of viral HA but not subtypes of HA strains. But these tests recognize human and avian influenza viral strains (H1N1, H2N3, H3N8, H4N6, H5N2, H6N2, H7N7, H8N4, H9N2, H10N7, H11N6, H12N6, H13N6, H14N5, H15N8, H16N3, H5N1, H5N6, H5N8, H7N1, N7 N7, and H7N9) as influenza type A viral infections (Tauns Inc.). By the results of these tests, and then if an antiviral therapy for influenza viral infection would be applied to patients. And then if an antiviral therapy is judged as not to be effective by the evaluation for the time of alleviation of fever in humans with influenza viral infections, further investigation for complications of viral infections, a new emerging viral infection using RIDTs for HA sub-strains, RT-PCR and/or viral cell culture, or mutant viruses resistant to antiviral drugs [13, 93]. In the pandemic phases 4–6, there may be many patients with influenza viral infection. It is very important to minimize the severe fatal disease from HPAI or LPAI infections and to select and send the patients with severe disease to the hospitals under the capacities for admission effectively by the triage between mild disease and severe disease. So this system may enable an early intervention of viral infections within 48 hours from onset and less numbers of patients with severe disease. It is not necessary to divide seasonal viral infection treatment from LPAI infection treatment except the necessity of special training and area for protection of widespread of EID using PPE. Like in the case with LPAI H6N1 virus in Taiwan [77], LPAI viral infections may be treated without identification in the circumstance of avian viral widespread among domestic birds. As one of the control points for pandemic preparedness, the candidate pandemic vaccine is desired and planned to be developed for prophylaxis and the most effective one of the control measures. The WHO has developed the influenza candidate vaccine viruses (CVVs) which are planned to be supplied to national authorities for pilot lot vaccine production, clinical trials, and other pandemic preparedness purposes based on their assessment of public health risk and need (contact at gisrs-whohq@who.int) [94]. Effective pandemic vaccines may be the most powerful measures for pandemic.

5. Conclusion

Pandemic is unpredictable, but sequential efforts to minimize and diminish the vulnerability of human public health from pandemic are desired in the world. Sentinel monitor and surveillance for endemic, epidemic, and pandemic potential is necessary for early detection of pandemic potential and pandemic preparedness planning. Sequential diagnosis and treatment from seasonal to avian influenza viruses adapted to humans may be beneficial in decreasing the risk of pandemic potential derived from zoonotic influenza virus infections. Preparations and developments of the candidate vaccine for the information following sequential monitor are necessary for the control against the phase of pre-pandemic and pandemic by avian influenza virus. The diverse of using several types of anti-influenza viral drugs with single and/or combinations for the pandemic infections would be desirable to be established as possible as a pandemic will be happen.

Conflict of interests

The author has no competing interests to declare.

Author details

Yuji Takemoto
Kamijyo Medical Office, Mori-machi, Izumiotsu City, Osaka Prefecture, Japan

*Address all correspondence to: y-t1@vesta.ocn.ne.jp

References

[1] Lambert T, Killoran K, Leedom Larson KR. Influenza C and influenza D Viruses. Swine Health Information Center and Center for Food Security and Public Health; 2016. Available from: http://www.cfsph.iastate.edu/pdf/shic-factsheet-influenza-cd

[2] Ali ST, Crowing BJ, EHY L, Fang VJ, Leung GM. Migration of influenza B epidemic with school closure, Hong Kong. Emerging Infectious Disease. 2018;**24**(11):2017-2073. DOI: 10.3021/eid2411.180612

[3] Abolnik C. A current review of avian influenza in pigeons and doves (Columbidae). Veterinary Microbiology. 2014;**170**:181-196. DOI: 10.1016/j.vetmic.2014.02.042

[4] Tong S, Li Y, Rivailler P, Conrardy C, Daa C, Chen LM, et al. A distinct lineage of influenza A virus from bats. Proceedings of the National Academy of Sciences of the United States of America. 2012;**109**:4269-4274. DOI: 10.1073/pnas.1116200109

[5] Tong S, Zhu X, Li Y, Shi M, Zhang J, Bourgeois M, et al. New world bats harbor diverse influenza A viruses. PLoS Pathogens. 2013;**9**:e1003657. DOI: 10.1371/journal.ppat.1003657

[6] Wiley DC, Skehel JJ. The structure and function of the hemagglutinin membrane glycoprotein of influenza virus. Annual Review of Biochemistry. 1987;**56**:3665-3394

[7] Kuiken T, Holmes EC, Mccauley J, Rimmelzwaan GF, William CS, Grenfell BT. Host species barriers to influenza virus infections. Science. 2006;**312**:394-397. DOI: 10.1126/science.1122818

[8] Nelson MI, Wentworth DE, Culhane MR, Vincent CA, LaPointe MP, Lin X, et al. Introductions and evolution of human-origin seasonal influenza A viruses in mutational swine populations. Journal of Virology. 2014;**88**:10110-10119. DOI: 10.1128/JVI.01080-14

[9] Korteweg C, Gu J. Pathology, molecular biology, and pathogenesis of avian influenza A (H5N1) infection in humans. The American Journal of Pathology. 2008;**172**(5):1155-1170. DOI: 10.2353/ajpath.2008.070791

[10] World Health Organization. Avian and Other Zoonotic Influenza. 2017. Available from: http://www.who.int/influenza/human_animal_interface/en/ [Accessed: 7 September 2017]

[11] World Health Organization. Influenza (Seasonal). Fact Sheet No. 211. Geneva: WHO; 2009. Available from: http://www.who.int/mediacentre/factsheets/fs211/en/index.html [Accessed: 9 December 2013]

[12] Centers for Disease Control and Prevention. Update. Isolation of avian influenza A (H5N1) Viruses from Humans—Hong Kong, 1997-1998. Morbidity and Mortality Weekly Report. 1998;**46**:1245-1247

[13] Takemoto Y, Asai T, Ikeszoe I, Yano T, Ichikawa M, Miyagawa S, et al. Clinical effects of oseltamivir, zanamivir, laninamivir and peramivir on seasonal influenza infection outpatients in Japan during the winter 2012-2013. Chemotherapy. 2013;**59**:373-378

[14] Claas EC, Osterhaus AD, van Beek R, De Jong JC, Rimmelzwaan GF, Senne DA, et al. Human influenza A H5N1 virus related to a highly pathogenic avian influenza virus. Lancet. 1998;**351**:472-477

[15] Yuen KY, Chan PK, Peiris M, Tsang DNC, Que TL, Cheung PT, et al. Clinical features and rapid viral diagnosis of human disease associated with avian

influenza A H5N1 virus. Lancet. 1998;**351**:467-471

[16] Available from: https://www.who.int/en/news-room/fact-sheets/detail/influenza-(avian-and-other-zoonotic)

[17] Connor RJ, Kawaoka Y, Webster RG, Paulson JC. Receptor specificity in human, avian, and equine H2 and H3 influenza virus isolates. Virology. 1994;**205**:17-23

[18] Baum LG, Paulson JC. Sialyloligosaccharides of the respiratory epithelium in the selection of human influenza virus receptor specificity. Acta Histochemica. Supplementband. 1990;**40**:35-38

[19] van Riel D, Munster VJ, de Wit E, Rimmelzwaan GF, Fouchier RA, Osterhaus AD, et al. H5N1 virus attachment to lower respiratory tract. Science. 2006;**312**:399

[20] Peiris JSM, Yu WC, Leung CW, Cheung CY, Ng WF, Nicholls JM, et al. Re-emergence of fatal human influenza A subtype H5N1 disease. Lancet. 2004;**363**:617-619

[21] Ungchusak K, Auewarakul P, Dowell SF, Kitphati R, Auwanit W, Puthavathana P, et al. Probable person-to-person transmission of avian influenza A (H5N1). The New England Journal of Medicine. 2005;**352**:333-340

[22] To KF, Chan PKS, Chan KF, Lee WK, Lam WY, Wong KF, et al. Pathology of fatal human infection associated with avian influenza A H5N1 virus. Journal of Medical Virology. 2001;**63**:242-246

[23] Gu J, Xie Z, Gao Z, Liu J, Korteweg C, Ye J, et al. H5N1 infection of the respiratory tract and beyond. Lancet. 2007;**370**:1137-1145

[24] Uiprasertkul MP, Puthavathana K, Sangsiriwut P, Pooruk P, Srisook K, Peiris M, et al. Influenza A H5N1 replication sites in humans. Emerging Infectious Diseases. 2005;**11**:1036-1041

[25] Uiprasertkul MP, Kitphati R, Puthavathana P, Kriwong R, Kongchanagul A, Ungchusak K, et al. Apoptosis and pathogenesis of avian influenza A (H5N1) virus in humans. Emerging Infectious Diseases. 2007;**13**:708-712

[26] Steinhauer DA. Role of hemagglutinin cleavage for the pathogenicity of influenza virus. Virology. 1999;**258**:1-20

[27] Katz JM, Lu X, Frace AM, Morken T, Zaki SR, Tumpey TM. Pathogenesis of and immunity to avian influenza A H5 viruses. Biomedicine & Pharmacotherapy. 2000;**54**:178-187

[28] Webster RG, Bean WJ, Gorman OT, Chambers TM, Kawaoka Y. Evolution and ecology of influenza A viruses. Microbiological Reviews. 1992;**56**:152-179

[29] Matrosovich M, Zhou N, Kawaoka Y, Webster R. The surface glycoproteins of H5 influenza viruses isolated from humans, chickens, and wild aquatic birds have distinguishable properties. Journal of Virology. 1999;**73**:1146-1155.30

[30] Hatta M, Gao P, Halfmann P, Kawaoka Y. Molecular basis for high virulence of Hong Kong H5N1 influenza A viruses. Science. 2001;**293**:1840-1842

[31] Taubenberger JK, Reid AH, Lourens RM, Wang R, Jin G, Fanning TG. Characterization of the 1918 influenza virus polymerase genes. Nature. 2005;**437**:889-893

[32] Chen W, Calvo PA, Malide D, Gibbs J, Schubert U, Bacik I, et al. A novel influenza A virus mitochondrial protein that induces cell death. Nature Medicine. 2001;**7**:1306-1312

[33] Obenauer JC, Denson J, Mehta PK, Su X, Mukatira S, Finkelstein DB, et al. Large-scale sequence analysis of avian influenza isolates. Science. 2006;**311**:1576-1580

[34] Kobasa D, Jones SM, Shinya K, Kash JC, Copps J, Ebihara H, et al. Aberrant innate immune response in lethal infection of macaques with the 1918 influenza virus. Nature. 2007;**445**:319-323

[35] Conenello GM, Zamarin D, Perrone LA, Tumpey T, Palese P. A single mutation in the PB1-F2 of H5N1 (HK/97) and 1918 influenza A viruses contributes to increased virulence. PLoS Pathogens. 2007;**3**:1414-1421

[36] Horimoto T, Kawaoka Y. Pandemic threat posed by avian influenza A viruses. Clinical Microbiology Reviews. 2001;**14**:129-149

[37] García-Sastre A, Egorov A, Matassov D, Brandt S, Levy DE, Durbin JE, et al. Influenza A virus lacking the NS1 gene replicates in interferon-deficient systems. Virology. 1998;**252**:324-330

[38] Seo SH, Hoffmann E, Webster RG. Lethal H5N1 influenza viruses escape host anti-viral cytokine responses. Nature Medicine. 2002;**8**:950-954

[39] Bender C, Hall H, Huang J, Klimov A, Cox N, Hay A, et al. Characterization of the surface proteins of influenza A (H5N1) viruses isolated from humans in 1997-1998. Virology. 1999;**254**:115-123

[40] de Jong MD, Simmons CP, Thanh TT, Hien VM, Smith GJ, Chau TN, et al. Fatal outcome of human influenza A (H5N1) is associated with high viral load and hypercytokinemia. Nature Medicine. 2006;**12**:1203-1207

[41] Li KS, Guan Y, Wang J, Smith GJ, Xu KM, Duan L, et al. Genesis of a highly pathogenic and potentially pandemic H5N1 influenza virus in eastern Asia. Nature. 2004;**430**:209-213

[42] Wang C, Lamb RA, Pinto LH. Activation of the M2 ion channel of influenza virus: A role for the transmembrane domain histidine residue. Biophysical Journal. 1995;**69**:1363-1371

[43] Smith GJ, Naipospos TS, Nguyen TD, de Jong MD, Vijaykrishna D, Usman TB, et al. Evolution and adaptation of H5N1 influenza virus in avian and human hosts in Indonesia and Vietnam. Virology. 2006;**350**:258-268

[44] Center for Disease Control and Prevention. Emergence of Avian Influenza A(H7N9) Virus Causing Severe Human Illness—China, February–April 2013. Morbidity and Mortality Weekly Report. 2013;**62**(18):366-371

[45] Wang C, Wang J, Su W, Gao S, Luo J, Zhang M, et al. Relationship between domestic and wild birds in live poultry market and a novel human H7N9 virus in China. The Journal of Infectious Diseases. 2014;**209**:34-37

[46] Available from: http://www.cidrap.umn.edu/sites/default/files/public/downloads/topics/cidrap_h7n9_update_051614_0.pdf

[47] Xu J et al. Reducing exposure to avian influenza H7N9. Lancet. 2013;**381**:1815-1816

[48] Murhekar M, Arima Y, Horby P, Vandemaele KA, Vong S, Zijian F, et al. Avian influenza A(H7N9) and the closure of live bird markets. Western Pacific Surveillance and Response Journal. 2013;**4**:4-7

[49] Mitigating the Impact of the New Influenza A (H1N1): Options for Public Health Measures. Manila: World Health Organization Regional Office for the Western Pacific; 2013

[50] Liu D, Shi W, Shi Y, Wang D, Xiao H, Li W, et al. Origin and diversity of novel avian influenza A H7N9 viruses causing human infection: phylogenetic, structural, and coalescent analyses. Lancet. 2013;**381**:1926-1932

[51] Kile JC, Ren R, Liu L, Greene CM, Roguski K, Luliano AD, et al. Morbidity and Mortality Weekly Report. 2017;**66**(35):928-932. Available from: https://www.cdc.gov/mmwr/volumes/66/wr/mm6635a2.htm?s_cid=mm6635a2_e

[52] Lam TT, Wang J, Shen Y, Zhou B, Duan L, Cheung CL, et al. The genesis and source of the H7N9 influenza viruses causing human infections in China. Nature. 2013;**502**:241-244

[53] Zhou J, Wang D, Gao R, Zhao B, Song J, Qi X, et al. Biological features of novel avian influenza A (H7N9) virus. Nature. 2013;**499**:500-503

[54] Kageyama T, Fujisaki S, Takashita E, Xu H, Yamada S, Uchida Y, et al. Genetic analysis of novel avian A(H7N9) influenza viruses isolated from patients in China, February to April 2013. Euro Surveillance. 2013;**18**:20453

[55] Massin P, van der Werf S, Naffakh N. Residue 627 of PB2 is a determinant of cold sensitivity in RNA replication of avian influenza viruses. Journal of Virology. 2001;**75**:5398-5404

[56] Mok CK, Lee HH, Lestra M, Nicholls JM, Chan MC, Sia SF, et al. Amino acid substitutions in polymerase basic protein 2 gene contribute to the pathogenicity of the novel A/H7N9 influenza virus in mammalian hosts. Journal of Virology. 2014;**88**:3568-3576

[57] Wu Y, Bi Y, Vavricka CJ, Sun X, Zhang Y, Gao F, et al. Characterization of two distinct neuraminidases from avian-origin human-infecting H7N9 influenza viruses. Cell Research. 2013;**23**:1347-1355

[58] Alexander DJ. A review of avian influenza in different bird species. Veterinary Microbiology. 2000;**74**:3-13

[59] Stegeman A, Bouman A, Elbers A, Jong M, Nodelijik G, Klerk F, et al. Avian influenza A virus (H7N7) epidemic in the Netherlands in 2003: Course of the epidemic and effectiveness of control measures. The Journal of Infectious Diseases. 2004;**190**:2088-2095

[60] Holle VB, Meijer A, Koopmans M, Jager CM. Human to human transmission of avian influenza A/H7N7, The Netherlands, 2003. Eurosurveillance. 2005;**10**:(12):264-268. Available from: https://www.eurosurveillance.org/content/10.2807/esm.10.12.00584-en

[61] Fouchier RA, Schneeberger PM, Rozendaal FW, Broekman JM, Kemink SAG, Munster V, et al. Avian influenza A (H7N7) virus associated with human conjunctivitis and a fatal case of acute respiratory distress syndrome. Proceedings of the National Academy of Sciences of the United States of America. 2004;**101**(5):1356-1361

[62] Capual I, Marangon S. Vaccination policy applied for the control of avian influenza in Italy. Developmental Biology. 2003;**114**:213-219

[63] Khan SU, Anderson B, Heil G, Laing S, Gray G. A systemic review and meta-analysis of the seropositive of influenza A (H9N2) infection among human. The Journal of Infectious Diseases. 2015;**212**:562-569. DOI: 10.1093/infdis/jiv109

[64] Lee DH, Swayne D, Sharma P, Rehmari SF, Wajid A, Suarez DL, et al. H9N2 low pathogenic avian influenza in Pakistan (2012-2015). Veterinary Record Open. 2016;**3**:e000171. DOI: 10.1136/vetreco-2016-000171

[65] Peiris M, Yuen KY, Leung CW, et al. Human infection with influenza H9N2. Lancet. 1999;**354**:916-917

[66] Pusch EA, Suarez DL. The multifaceted zoonotic risk of H9N2 avian influenza. Journal of Veterinary Science. 2018;**5**:82. DOI: 10.3390/vetsci5040082

[67] Pulliam JR, Dushoff JG, Levin SA, Dobson AP. Epidemic enhancement in partially immune populations. PLoS One. 2007;**2**:e165

[68] Guan Y, Shortridge KF, Krauss S, Webster RG. Molecular characterization of H9N2 influenza viruses: Were they the donors of the "internal" genes of H5N1 viruses in Hong Kong? Proceedings of the National Academy of Sciences of the United States of America. 1999;**96**:9363-9367

[69] Chen H, Yuan H, Gao R, et al. Clinical and epidemiological characteristics of a fatal case of avian influenza A H10N8 virus infection: a descriptive study. Lancet. 2014;**383**:714-721

[70] OIE. World Organisation for Animal Health. 2017. Available from: http://www.oie.int/animal-health-in-the-world/update-on-avian-influenza/ [Accessed: 7 November 2017]

[71] World Health Organization. Weekly Epidemiological Record Relevpidmiologique Hebdomadaire, Vol. 92. 2017. pp. 453-476. Available from: http://www.who.int/wer

[72] Zhang Z, Li R, Jiang L, Xiong C, Chen Y, Zhao G, et al. The complexity of human infected AIV H5N6 isolated from China. BMC Infectious Diseases. 2016;**16**(1):600

[73] Yang L, Zhu W, Li X, Bo H, Zhang Y, Zou S, et al. Genesis and dissemination of highly pathogenic H5N6 avian influenza viruses. Journal of Virology. 2017;**91**(5):129-144

[74] Avian Influenza A (H7N2) in Cats in Animal Shelter in NY; One Human Infection. CDC24/7. Available from: https://www.cdc.gov/flu/spotlights/avian-influenza-cats.htm

[75] Belser JA, Blixt O, Chen LM, Pappas C, Maines TR, Hoeven NV, et al. Contemporary North American influenza H7 viruses possess human receptor specificity: Implications for virus transmissibility. Proceedings of the National Academy of Sciences of the United States of America. 2008;**105**(21):7558-7563

[76] Tweed SA, Skowronski DM, David ST, Larder A, Petric M, Lees W, et al. Human illness from avian influenza H7N3, British Columbia. Emerging Infectious Diseases. 2004;**10**(12):2196-2199. DOI: 10.3201/eid1012.040961

[77] Center for Infectious Disease Research and Policy (CIDRP). Taiwan Reports First in Human H6N1 Infection. 2013. Available from: http://www.cidrap.umn.edu/news-perspective/2013/06/taiwan-reports-first-human-h6n1-infection

[78] Vries RP, Tzarum NT, Peng W, Tompson AI, Wickramashinghe IS, Pena AT, et al. A single mutation in Taiwanese H6N1 influenza hemagglutinin switches binding to human type receptors. EMBO Molecular Medicine. 2017;**9**:1314-1325

[79] Arzey GG, Kirkland PD, Arzey KE, Frost M, Maywood P, Conaty S, et al. Influenza virus A (H10N7) in chickens and poultry abattoir workers, Australia. Emerging Infectious Disease. 2012;**8**(5). Available from: https://wwwnc.cdc.gov/eid/article/18/5/11-1852_article

[80] Olsen CW, Brown I, Easterday BC, Van Reeth K. Swine influenza. In: Straw B, D'Allaire S, Zimmerman J, Taylor D, editors. Diseases of Swine. 9th ed. Iowa, USA: Iowa State University Press; 2006. pp. 469-482. Available from: https://www.bookdepository.com/Diseases-Swine-David-J-Taylor/9780813817033

[81] Yu H, Zhang PC, Zhou YJ, Li GX, Pan J, Yan LP, et al. Isolation and genetic characterization of avian–like H1N1 and novel reassortant H1N2 influenza viruses from pigs in China. Biochemical and Biophysical Research Communications. 2009;**21**:278-283. DOI: 10.1016/j.bbrc.2009.05.056

[82] Liang H, Lam TTY, Fan X, Chen X, Zeng Y, Zhou J, et al. Expansion of genotypic diversity and establishment of 2009 H1N1 pandemic-origin internal genes in pigs in China. Journal of Virology;**2014, 88**:10864-10874. DOI: 10.1128/JVI.01327-14

[83] Horimoto KI, Shi J, Wang X, Tagawa YS, Ito M, Murakami K, et al. Development of a influenza diagnostic kit specific for the H7 subtype. Frontiers in Microbiology. 2018;**9**:1346

[84] Avian Influenza and Human Pandemic Influenza. Summary Report; 7-9 November 2005; Geneva, Switzerland. 2005

[85] WHO Library Global Epidemiological Surveillance Standards for Influenza. Available from: https://www.who.int/influenza/resources/documents/WHO_Epidemiological_Influenza_Surveillance_Standards_2014.pdf?ua=1

[86] WHO. Pandemic Influenza Preparedness and Response: A WHO Guidance Document. Available from: https://www.ncbi.nlm.nih.gov/books/NBK143061/

[87] WHO. Influenza (Avian and Other Zoonotic). 2018. Available from: https://www.who.int/news-room/fact-sheets/detail/influenza-(avian-and-other-zoonotic)

[88] WHO. International Food Safety Authorities Network (INFOSAN) Highly Pathogenic H5N1 Avian Influenza Outbreaks in Poultry and in Humans: Food Safety Implications. 2005. Available from: https://www.who.int/foodsafety/fs_management/No_07_AI_Nov05_en.pdf?ua=1

[89] Ungchusak K, Auewarakul P, Dowell SF, Kitphati R, Auwanit W, Puthavathana P, et al. Probable person-to-person transmission of avian influenza A (H5N1). The New England Journal of Medicine. 2005;**352**(4):333-340. DOI: 10.1056/NEMJMoa044021

[90] WHO. Pandemic Influenza Preparedness and Response: A WHO Guidance Document. 4. The WHO Pandemic Phase

[91] Muthuri SG, Myles PJ, Venkatesan S, Leonardi-Bee J, Nguyen-Van-Tam J. Impact of neuraminidase inhibitor treatment on outcomes of public health importance during the 2009-2010 influenza A (H1N1) pandemic: A systematic review and meta-analysis in hospitalised patients. The Journal of Infectious Diseases. 2013;**207**:553-563

[92] Noshi T, Kitano M, Taniguchi K, Yamamoto A, Omoto S, Baba K, et al. In vitro characterization of baloxavir acid, a first-in-class cap-dependent endonuclease inhibitor of the influenza virus polymerase PA unit. Antiviral Research. 2018;**160**:109-117

[93] Takemoto Y. Therapeutic approach for seasonal influenza and pandemic. IntechOpen book series Infectious Disease. In: Influenza: Therapeutics and Challenges. Vol. 1. 2018. pp. 133-150

[94] WHO. Antigenic and Genetic Characteristics of Zoonotic Influenza Viruses and Candidate Vaccine Viruses Developed for Potential Use in Human Vaccines. 2018. pp. 1-13. Available from: https://www.who.int/influenza/vaccines/virus/characteristics_virus_vaccines/en/

Section 3

Measles - The Knowns and Unknowns

Chapter 8

Measles in Developing Countries

Anyebe Onoja and Oluwaseyi Ajagbe

Abstract

Measles is a major childhood problem which causes significant illness, death and disability. It infects approximately 40 million people resulting in nearly 1 million deaths annually in developing countries. Measles virus accounts for 44% of total deaths among children that are less than 15 years of age. Highest mortality occurs among children living in poor communities especially in areas that are overcrowded, and where there is malnutrition and vaccination coverage is low. Most of the measles infections in the world are recorded in developing countries of Africa and Asia. Endemic areas are largely confined to the tropics, where transmission increases after rainy season. Inability to effectively immunize most children in this area has hampered global measles mortality reduction initiatives and reduction of under-five child mortality. Although, this was initially scheduled to have been met by 2015, recent WHO resolution called for measles elimination in the African Region by 2020. It is not certain that this will be met; hence the need for coordinated and strategic mass vaccination efforts to target unimmunized children in these regions.

Keywords: measles virus, genotypes, immunization, vaccination, coverage, Africa

1. Introduction

Measles is a serious medical problem in Africa, Latin America, Europe, southeast Asia and eastern Mediterranean [1]. During the pre-vaccine era, 130 million measles cases occurred annually worldwide, and it was the leading cause of childhood deaths [2]. In Africa, about 13 million cases and 650,000 deaths occur annually, with sub-Saharan Africa having the highest morbidity and mortality [3]. In 2018, many developing countries reportedly confirmed measles through laboratory testing with high incidence rates. In AFRO region, Liberia confirmed 218 cases with 412.24% incidence rate. Similarly, Libya confirmed 286 cases with 98.84% incidence rate, Burkina Fasso confirmed 567 cases with 84.2% incidence rate and the southern part of the continent was not left out as Uganda confirmed 531 cases in the laboratory with incidence rate of 65.83%. In the Western Pacific region, Philippines confirmed 1677 cases with incidence rate of 118.5% while Malaysia confirmed 1374 cases with incidence rate of 80.35% [4]. In EURO region, Albania confirmed 1290 cases with incidence rate of 477.05%, Georgia reported 1091 laboratory confirmed cases with 374.74% incidence rate and Kyrgyzstan confirmed 376 cases in the laboratory with 75.22% incidence rate. In EMRO, Afghanistan reported 1846 laboratory confirmed cases with 62.64% incidence rate, Saudi Arabia reported 833 laboratory confirmed cases with 29.99% and 793 laboratory confirmed cases in Yemen with incidence rate of 344.36%. Venezuela in AMRO confirmed 5525 cases in the laboratory with an incidence rate of 23.03% [4].

Despite the comprehensive WHO and United Nations International Children Emergency Fund's (UNICEF's) measles-reduction strategy, and partnership of international organizations for measles mortality reduction, certain countries continue to face recurrent epidemics [5]. The optimal age for infantile measles vaccination is an important since maternal antibodies may neutralize the vaccine antigen before specific immune response develops. Delaying vaccination on the other hand may increase risk of complicated disease [6]. Measles vaccine effectiveness is 84% when administered at 9–11 months of age and 93% when given at ≥12 months of age [7]. First dose of measles-containing vaccine (MCV1) given at 9 months of age was introduced into the Expanded Programme on Immunization (EPI) in 1977 [8]. Since >93–95% population immunity is required to prevent measles epidemics, the WHO recommends all children receive two doses of measles vaccine [9]. In Nigeria just like in many developing countries, children are given monovalent measles vaccine at 9 months of age in the EPI [10]. In 2010 and continuing through 2014, DRC experienced the largest nationwide measles outbreak in Africa [11–13]. DRC is a key country for regional elimination efforts because of its large population, central location with nine international borders, and persistent reservoir of circulating measles viruses [14]. The Reaching Every District (RED) approach to strengthening immunization services has been implemented beginning in some developing countries like Democratic Republic of Congo (DRC). A second opportunity for measles vaccination, nationwide measles supplementary immunization activities (SIAs) using a phased approach intended to cover the country every 3 years [15].

2. Epidemiology and immunization

2.1 Measles virus detection strategies and sero-surveillance in Africa

Following a successful polio laboratory platform, The Global Measles and Rubella Laboratory Network (GMRLN) was developed. As at 2018, there are presently 723 laboratories established in 164 countries. It was proposed that in all districts in WHO AFRO surveillance performance should target ≥2 cases of non-measles febrile rash illness per 100,000 population and ≥1 suspected measles case investigated with blood specimens in ≥80% of districts [16]. Case-based surveillance with laboratory confirmation of suspected measles cases is in place in many developing countries. Integrated Disease Surveillance and Response (IDSR) was established for aggregate reporting of 18 infectious diseases, including measles. Through the IDSR, aggregate numbers of suspected measles cases and deaths are reported weekly from districts to national level. Through measles case-based surveillance, suspected measles cases were investigated using case investigation form and laboratory testing of blood specimen. Specimens are tested using standard enzyme-linked immunosorbent assays for measles-specific immunoglobulin M (IgM) antibodies. Suspected measles case was defined as an illness with maculopapular rash and fever and one or more symptoms of cough, coryza or conjunctivitis, or where clinician suspects measles. Laboratory-confirmed measles case on the other hand is defined as suspected measles case with positive laboratory test result for measles specific IgM in the absence of measles vaccination within 30 days of specimen collection. An epidemiologically-linked case is suspected measles case having contact (or living in same district) with laboratory-confirmed measles case whose rash onset was within preceding 30 days. Clinically-compatible case is suspected measles case without laboratory test result or established epidemiological link. PCR detection is carried out in specific laboratories with technology for confirm hemagglutinin (H) and nucleoprotein (NP) gene of measles virus.

2.2 Circulating genotypes and clades in Africa

Measles virus is monotypic; however, genetic variations occur in the H and NP genes. Currently, the WHO recognizes 8 clades, A-H which consists of 24 genotypes and an additional provisional genotype, D11. Clades B, C, D, G and H each contain multiple genotypes (B1-3, C1-2, D1-10, G1-3 and H1-2) while clades A, E and F each contain single genotype (A, E and F) respectively [17, 18]. Epidemiological findings reveal circulation of several genotypes in Africa. Genotype A has been detected in South America, parts of China and South Africa over the last 40 years [19], and recently in a 3 year old child in Nigeria West Africa [20]. The most endemic genotype circulating in Africa is B3. Studies have shown clade B to be endemic in sub-Saharan Africa [21] with B3 genotype reported in Ghana, Gambia, Nigeria, Libya and Tunisia [20, 22, 23]. The measles viruses isolated in 1983 from Yaoundé, Cameroon, were designated as B1 genotype. However, in 2001 viruses belonging to B3 genotype were found in the country. B3 genotype has been reported in the Gambia. The B3 genotype (2001) in Cameroon were related to B3.1 subgroup, whereas the Gambian (1993) isolates corresponded to B3.2 subgroup. Geographical distribution for period 1993–2001 of these two viruses shows that B3.1 is found from Sudan to Nigeria and Ghana extending to Cameroon, whereas B3.2 genotype is found in West Africa. In Nigeria and Ghana, the viruses co-circulate [3, 14]. Nucleotide sequence analysis show strains from Senegal clustered in B3.1 and B3.3 sub-genotypes. Measles virus detected in Tunisia and Libya from 2002 to 2009 belonged to genotype B3. Viruses isolated from 2002 to 2007 and 2009 were subtype B3.1. Seven of isolates during 2008 and 2009 epidemic were divergent from the B3 isolates and can represent a new subtype of genotype B3 [21]. B3 strain circulates in Addis Ababa, Bahir Dar and possibly elsewhere in Ethiopia [24]. In a 2014 outbreak among refugees from Central African Republic in Cameroon, the genotype B3 found were similar to those circulating in Northern Cameroon in 2010–2011 [25]. Clade B viruses is reported to be endemic in central and western parts of sub-Saharan Africa while genotypes D2 and D4 has been continually detected in southern and eastern parts of Africa. D10 in Uganda is represented by Clade MVi/Kampala. UGA/51.00.1 with accession number AY923185.1. Genotype C2 is found to circulate widely in northern Africa [17, 26–28].

2.3 MV complications in developing countries

Measles is characterized by fever of 38°C or more; maculopapular rash of 3 days or more; with one or combination of coryza, cough, conjunctivitis and Koplik spots in the oral mucosa of measles' victims [29]. Mortality rates can exceed 10% in parts of the developing world. Sequela of measles includes giant cell pneumonia, inclusion body encephalitis and sub-acute sclerosing pan encephalitis [SSPE] [30]. A study carried out in the largest children's hospital in Ibadan-Nigeria in West Africa observed several complications ranging from bronchopneumonia (60%), heart failure (12%), gastroenteritis (11%), protein losing malnutrition (8%), encephalitis (5%), croup (2%) and dehydration (2%) [10], whereas bacterial complication is the usual cause of death when measles kills malnourished children [31].

2.4 Vaccination and herd immunity

After routine and catch-up vaccinations in 2005 and 2006, as well as follow-up vaccination by 2008 in Nigeria, remarkable level of protection was observed in children. This is attributed to immunological dynamics which is an after-effect of these campaigns [32]. Herd immunity varies between heterogeneous populations in developing countries. Nigeria is the most populous country in Africa with a population of over 160million. In an assessment of immune status carried out in 2014, herd immunity against measles was 66.8% in Kano State and 73.0% in Ibadan, Oyo State. These are two largely different populations in the north and southern respectively [33]. When history of measles was compared with level of immunity, a significant association was observed between those who had measles and who had protective immunity. There was strong correlation between malnutrition and immune level, a lot of malnourished children who were vaccinated were not protected [33].

2.5 Measles vaccination coverage in Africa

Strategies based on vaccination program have been implemented in order to reduce measles mortality. In 2008, countries in the WHO African Region adopted measles pre-elimination goal to be achieved by the end of 2012. Target was to achieve >98% reduction in estimated regional measles mortality. The goal was to have national measles incidence of <5 cases per 1,000,000 population per year, achieve >90% national coverage with MCV1 with >80% MCV1 coverage target. For SIAs, MCV coverage >95% was targeted in all districts [16]. In the WHO regions, highest percentage of reduction was in Eastern Mediterranean (90%) and African (89%) regions, accounting for 16 and 63% of global reduction [34, 35]. Relatively high measles vaccination in southern Nigeria in West Africa can be attributed to high level of literacy and awareness created by free use of mass media to disseminate information on vaccination activities, without fear of intimidation [33]. The Global Vaccine Action Plan (GVAP) set out a target of reaching 80% coverage with all vaccines including measles vaccine in all districts by 2020 [36]. Health policy decision-making based on spatially heterogeneous vaccination has resulted in shift from pursuing coverage targets at national-level to ensuring high coverage levels evenly distributed across provinces or districts [37]. While this likely represents a more effective strategy over targeting country-level goals, administrative area summaries may still mask important geographical inequities in coverage [38].

2.6 Challenges of measles immunization in resource-limited settings

Vaccination history of children is not documented in hospital's records because many people do not properly keep children's/wards' vaccination records. This is coupled with high illiteracy level found in many developing countries [32]. Many people present as emergencies upon admission, at which point their parents cared less about vaccination status because they were overwhelmed by anxiety. There is need for enhanced comprehensive national vaccination campaigns with intense community engagement and diligent health workers including large number of ad-hoc staff. Weak government support across all levels is responsible for poor surveillance activities hence, their inability to detect new cases. Awareness creation should be intensified to inform concerned citizens about the essence and time of vaccination.

Ability to produce vaccines is a major setback for developing countries. Japan International Cooperation Agency (JICA) is currently supporting transfer of a Measles-Rubella vaccine manufacturing technology to Polyvac® in Vietnam, following the precedent set by multiple previous successful projects. Transfer of an oral polio vaccine (OPV) technology from Biken Co., Ltd. to Bio Farma in Indonesia was pivotal in the global polio eradication efforts. JICA supports UNICEF supply of vaccine cold chain equipment to India, Afghanistan, Angola, Liberia, Zambia and Zimbabwe which has significantly overcome the problem of vaccine failure resulting from inability of most immunization officers to maintain cold chain in remote areas.

Government bodies responsible for ensuring safety and effectiveness of vaccines face serious challenges when protecting the public from harm once the products are used in uncontrolled, real world context [39–41]. Regulations have been moving towards an approach that takes into account the full lifecycle of the vaccine. While this shift has been very slow in countries like Canada, there have been further calls for changes on how regulators safeguard public health and public healthcare resources [42]. This approaches are a far cry from the reality on ground in developing countries, because they utilize whatever vaccines are supplied by donor agencies or vendors who have passed through government's registration processes.

Most countries grapple with unreliable immunization service funding. But in spite of active measles vaccination efforts in several developing countries, re-emergence of measles continues to occur [33]. An interplay of several factors affect immunization. These factors include break in cold-chain of measles vaccine due to long distance to vaccination centers, history of measles, intercurrent infections and malnutrition. In both developing and industrialized countries, loss of public confidence in vaccine due to real or spurious links to adverse events can curtail or even halt immunization activities. This is similar to reports about polio vaccine laced with sterilizing agents which led to decline in vaccination uptake in northern Nigeria. Despite the scientific evidence refuting links between the measles-mumps-rubella (MMR) vaccine and autism, there has been decline in coverage in some countries as a result of this. Measles is making a comeback in several industrialized countries, including Austria, Italy and the United Kingdom. This can be attributed to presence of migrants and refugees from developing countries especially those who are biased against vaccines in light spurious or religious sentiments.

Masking of geographical inequalities in vaccination because of poor administrative summaries is a big problem. Spatial clustering of unvaccinated children sustains disease transmission, even when high overall vaccination coverage is achieved. Continued measles virus circulation occurs as a result of missing age cohorts during routine vaccination. Access to high quality vaccines is important however, there is limited expertise to review technical product information in vaccine regulatory dossiers hence the inability to effectively register and supply vaccines in many developing countries. They lack appropriate expertise and certified personnel to perform good manufacturing practice (GMP) inspections leading to lengthy registration/review process and delays in vaccine registration even in emergency situations. Worrisome is the fact that there is limited compliance with good clinical practice standards for some clinical trials. Therefore, improving vaccine supply chain in developing countries is very important. A review of existing data shows freeze exposure occurred in 18–67% of vaccine shipments throughout various stages of storage. Also, heat denatures vaccines when cold chain is not maintained. Such may reduce vaccine potency, ultimately supplying potentially less-effective vaccines.

2.7 Sourcing of vaccines

The developing countries vaccine manufacturers' network (DCVMN) is a public health driven, international alliance of manufacturers trying to strengthen vaccine supply through information and professional training programs, technology improvements, innovative vaccine research and development, encouraging transfer initiatives, to improve availability of safe, effective and affordable vaccines. Three goals were proposed for vaccines. First, to ensure uninterrupted supply of affordable and suitable vaccines for GAVI. Second, improve market dynamics information and expertise to solve vaccine access challenges. Third, strengthening global health and manufacturers' partnerships to enable better alignment of goals, alignment with global strategy and coordination of internal investments [43].

2.8 Negative impact of population explosion

Civil unrest is common in developing countries and this has led to migration of millions of people. There is increased movement by land, air and sea. In Northern Nigeria, activities of Boko Haram terrorist have caused several families to abandon their homelands and converge on Internally Displaced Peoples camps where health care services are poor and even non-existent in some cases. Many children are born in these camps, but vaccination activities may not be sustained at the desired national vaccination level. Wars and famines or other natural disasters increase mortality due to measles. In 2000, measles was responsible for 22% of deaths in children less than 5 years of age and 17% of deaths in children aged 5–14 years in Ethiopia [44]. Increased air travel by people within some regions in developing countries has been reported. For local flights, cabin air flow may not be as reliable a barrier to the spread of measles virus. Several measles reports, including index cases and apparent secondary cases on flights, have been reported in which transmission on board the aircraft appeared likely and which included seating information for both index (primary) and secondary case [45].

3. Conclusion

Regulations for safety and effectiveness of vaccines in the uncontrolled, real world context should be strengthened in developing countries. Perhaps the set of ethical considerations when fully operational in developed countries will be applied to them also. The World Health Assembly established 3 milestones towards eradication of measles. They intend to increase routine coverage with MCV1 by more than 90% nationally and more than 80% in every district; reduce and maintain annual measles incidence to less than 5 cases per million; and reduce estimated measles mortality by more than 95%. Based on current trends of measles vaccination coverage and incidence, and report of the strategic review, the WHO Strategic Advisory Group of Experts on Immunization (SAGE) concluded that the 2015 global milestones and measles elimination goals were not achieved because immunization coverage gaps exist. SAGE recommended focus on improving immunization and surveillance systems to ensure gains made thus far in measles control can be sustained. The situation in developing countries requires serious attention and strict compliance by stakeholders to ensure goals are met.

Conflict of interest

We declare that there is no conflict of interest.

Author details

Anyebe Onoja[1]* and Oluwaseyi Ajagbe[2]

1 Department of Virology, College of Medicine, University of Ibadan, Nigeria

2 Faculty of Veterinary Medicine, University of Abuja, Nigeria

*Address all correspondence to: bernardonoja@yahoo.com

References

[1] World Health Organization. Reported Measles Cases and Incidence Rates by WHO Member States 2010 and 2011. WHO Factsheet; 2011. Available from: http://www.who.int/immunization_monitoring/diseases/measlesreportedcasesbycountry.pdf

[2] World Health Organization. Response to Measles Outbreaks in Measles Mortality Reduction Settings. WHO/IVB/09.03; Geneva: The Organization; 2009

[3] Muller CP, Hanses F, Troung A, Ammerhan WO, Ikusika W, Adu F. Molecular epidemiology of Nigerian and Ghanaian measles virus isolates reveals a genotype circulating widely in western and central Africa. The Journal of General Virology. 1999;**80**(4):871-877. DOI: 10.1099/0022-1317-80-4-871

[4] WHO. Reported Measles Cases and Incidence Rates by WHO Member States, as of 09 November 2018; 2018

[5] Grais RF, Dubray C, Gerstl S, Guthmann JP, Djibo A, Nargaye KD, et al. Unacceptably high mortality related to measles epidemics in Niger, Nigeria and Chad. PLoS Medicine. 2007;**4**(1):e16. DOI: 10.1371/journal.pmed.0040016

[6] Gagneur A, Pinquier D, Aubert M, Balu L, Brissaud O, De Pontual L, et al. Kinetics of decline of maternal measles virus-neutralizing antibodies in sera of infants in France in 2006. Clinical and Vaccine Immunology. 2008;**15**(12):1845-1850. DOI: 10.1128/CVI.00229-08

[7] Ma-Disu M. Role of nongovernmental agencies in vaccine delivery. Reviews of Infectious Diseases. 1989;**11**(Supplement 3): 5646-5648. DOI: 10.1093/clinids/11.supplement_3.s646

[8] Uzicanin A, Zimmerman L. Field effectiveness of live attenuated measles-containing vaccines: A review of published literature. The Journal of Infectious Diseases. 2011;**204**(Suppl 1): S13348. DOI: 10.1093/infdis/jir102

[9] World Health Organization. Measles vaccines: WHO position paper. Weekly Epidemiological Record. 2009;**84**(35):349-360

[10] Onoja AB, Adeniji AJ, Faneye A. Measles complications in a Nigerian hospital setting. Clinical Reviews and Opinions. 2013;**5**(2):18-23. DOI: 10.5897/CRO12.008

[11] Grout L, Minetti A, Hurtado N, François G, Fermon F, Chatelain A, et al. Measles in Democratic Republic of Congo: An outbreak description from Katanga, 2010-2011. BMC Infectious Diseases. 2013;**13**:232. DOI: 10.1186/1471-2334-13-232

[12] WHO. Effective Vaccine Management Assessments for 57 GAVI Countries: Average Score of Principal, Sub-National Local District and Service Point Level. Final Report for IRC Gavi. Available from: http://www.gavi.org/Library/GAVI../IRC../Final-Report-for-IRC-Nov-2014/

[13] Mancini S, Coldiron ME, Ronsse CA, Ilunga BKI, Porten K, Grais RF. Description of a large measles epidemic in Democratic Republic of Congo, 2010-2013. Conflict and Health. 2014;**8**:9. DOI: 10.1186/1752-1505-8-9

[14] Kremer JR, Nkwembe E, Bola Oyefolu AO, et al. Measles virus strain diversity, Nigeria and Democratic Republic of the Congo. Emerging Infectious Diseases. 2010;**16**(11):1724-1730. DOI: 10.3201/eid1611.100777

[15] Ministry of Public Health Expanded Programme on Immunization. Democratic Republic of the Congo Measles Control Plan 2013-2015.

Kinshasa, Democratic Republic of the Congo; 2012

[16] World Health Organization. Report of the Second Meeting of the African Regional Measles Technical Advisory Group (TAG), Recommendations. Addis Ababa, Ethiopia: World Health Organization, Regional Office for Africa; 2008. Available from: http://www.afro.who.int/index.php?option=com_docman&task=doc_download&gid=3616

[17] World Health Organization. Nomenclature for describing the genetic characteristics of wild-type measles viruses. Part 1. Weekly Epidemiological Record. 2001;**76**(32):242-247

[18] Rota PA, Bellini WJ. Update on the global distribution of genotypes of wild type measles viruses. The Journal of Infectious Diseases. 2003;**187**(Suppl 1): S270-S276. DOI: 10.1086/368042

[19] Riddell MA, Rota JS, Rota PA. Review of the temporal and geographical distribution of measles virus genotypes in the prevaccine and postvaccine eras. Virology Journal. 2005;**2**:87. DOI: 10.1186/1743-422X-2-87

[20] Faneye AO, Adeniji JA, Motayo BO. Genetic analysis of measles virus nucleocapsid gene identifies measles virus isolate of close similarity to clade A viruses from Nigeria. F1000Research. 2018;**7**:155. DOI: 10.12688/f1000research.13565.1

[21] Haddad-Boubaker S, Rezq M, Smeo MN, Ben Yahia A, Abudher A, Slim A, et al. Genetic characterization of clade B measles viruses isolated in Tunisia and Libya 2002-2009 and a proposed new subtype within the B3 genotype. Virus Research. 2010;**153**(2):258-264. DOI: 10.1016/j.virusres.2010.08.011

[22] Dia N, Fall A, Rouguiyatou K, Amary Fall A, Kiori DE, Goudiaby DG, et al. Epidemiology and genetic characterization of measles strains in Senegal, 2004-2013. PLoS One. 2015;**10**(5):e0121704. DOI: 10.1371/journal.pone.0121704

[23] Rota PA, Brown K, Mankertz A, et al. Global distribution of measles genotypes and measles molecular epidemiology. The Journal of Infectious Diseases. 2011;**204**(S1):S514-S523. DOI: 10.1093/infdis/jir118

[24] Lemma E, Smit SB, Beyene B, Nigatu W, Babaniyi OA. Genetic characterization and progression of B3 measles genotype in Ethiopia: A study of five measles outbreak cases. Ethiopian Medical Journal. 2008;**46**(1):79-85

[25] Ndombo P, Ndze V, Mbarga F, Anderson R, Acho A, Chia E, et al. Molecular characterisation of measles virus strains among refugees from Central African Republic in Cameroon in 2014. Epidemiology and Infection. 2018;**146**(3):319-323. DOI: 10.1017/S0950268817002990

[26] Kres S, Vadas E, Whistler T. Sequence analysis of the nucleocapsid gene of measles virus isolates from South Africa identifies a new genotype. The Journal of General Virology. 1997;**78**(7):1581-1587. DOI: 10.1099/0022-1317-78-7-1581

[27] WHO. New genotype of measles virus and update on global distribution of measles genotypes. Weekly Epidemiological Record. 2005;**80**(40):347-351

[28] Muwonge A, Nanyuja M, Rota PA, et al. New measles genotype, Uganda. Emerging Infectious Diseases. 2005;**11**(10):1522-1526. DOI: 10.3201/eid1110.050431

[29] Steichen O, Dautheville S. Koplik spots in early measles. CMAJ. 2009;**180**(5):583. DOI: 10.1503/cmaj.080724

[30] Holzmann H, Hengel H, Tenbusch M, Doerr H. Eradication of measles: Remaining challenges. Medical Microbiology and Immunology. 2016;**205**(3):201-208. DOI: 10.1007/s00430-016-0451-4

[31] White DO, Fenner FJ. Medical Virology. 4th ed. San Diego, California: Academic Press, a division of Harcourt Brace and Company; 1994. pp. 461-465

[32] Onoja AB, Adeniji AJ. Kinetics of measles antibody by haemagglutination inhibition assay in children in south-west and north-central Nigerian state. International Journal of Infectious Diseases. 2013;**17**(7):552-555. DOI: 10.1016/j.ijid.2013.02.001

[33] Onoja AB, Hamid KM, Adeniji JA, Mukhtar MD. Implication of vaccination on measles reduction and elimination in Nigeria. African Journal of Medicine and Medical Sciences. 2014;**43**(Suppl 1): 73-78

[34] CDC. Progress in global measles control and mortality reduction, 2000-2007. Morbidity and Mortality Weekly Report. 2008;**57**(48):1303-1306

[35] Zarocostas J. Mortality from measles fell by 91% in Africa from 2000 to 2006. BMJ. 2007;**335**(7631):1173. DOI: 10.1136/bmj.39419.393275.DB

[36] Lessler J, Metcalf CJE, Grais RF, Luquero FJ, Cummings DAT, Grenfell BT. Measuring the performance of vaccination programs using cross-sectional surveys: A likelihood framework and retrospective analysis. PLoS Medicine. 2011;**8**(10):e1001110. DOI: 10.1371/journal.pmed.1001110

[37] WHO. Global Vaccine Action Plan 2011-2020. 2013. Available from: http://www.who.int/immunization/global_vaccine_action_plan/en/

[38] Takahashi S, Metcalf CJE, Ferrari MJ, Tatem AJ, Lessler J. The geography of measles vaccination in the African Great Lakes region. Nature Communications. 2017;**8**:15585. DOI: 10.1038/ncomms15585

[39] Arlett P, Portier G, de Lisa R, Blake K, Wathion N, Dogne J-M, et al. Proactively managing the risk of marketed drugs: Experience with the EMA pharmacovigilance risk assessment committee. Nature Reviews Drug Discovery. 2014;**13**:395-397. DOI: 10.1038/nrd3713-c1

[40] Health Canada. Lifecycle Approach Model. Health Products and Food Regulatory Modernization. 2012. Available from: http://www.hc-sc.gc.ca/ahc-asc/activit/strateg/mod/ini/index-eng.php

[41] Institute of Medicine. Ethical and Scientific Issues in Studying the Safety of Approved Drugs. Washington, DC: The National Academies Press; 2012

[42] Standing Senate Committtee on Social Affairs, Science and Technology. Prescription Pharmaceuticals in Canada Post-Approval Monitoring of Safety and Effectiveness. Ottawa: Standing Senate Committtee on Social Affairs, Science and Technology; 2013

[43] Pagliusi S, Jain R, Suri RK. Vaccines, our shared responsibilities. Vaccine. 2015;**33**:2197-2202. DOI: 10.1016/j.vaccine.2015.02.065

[44] Salama P, Assefa F, Talley L, Spiegel P, van Der Veen A, Gotway CA. Malnutrition, measles, mortality, and the humanitarian response during a famine in Ethiopia. Journal of the American Medical Association. 2001;**286**:563-571. DOI: 10.1001/jama.286.5.563

[45] Edelson PJ. Patterns of measles transmission among airplane travellers. Travel Medicine and Infectious Disease. 2012;**10**(5-6):230-235. DOI: 10.1016/j.tmaid.2012.10.003

Chapter 9

Estimation of Measles Immunization Coverage in Guwahati by Ranked Set Sampling

Vivek Verma and Dilip C. Nath

Abstract

In order to study the efficacy of the ranked set sampling (RSS), as an alternative procedure, for estimation of the proportion of children aged 12–23 immunized against measles vaccine, a study is conducted in slum and non-slum regions of Guwahati, the capital of Assam, India. The RSS-based approach in the cases of both perfect and imperfect rankings is compared with its counterpart simple random sampling (SRS). The results revealed that estimates based on RSS with set size (4) are very close to Census report for Assam (2012) and has less variability than the SRS estimator. RSS-based estimates for different choices of probability of ranking error (ρ) are not only more accurate but are more precise and efficient than the SRS procedure, and also suggest that a the procedure of RSS better than the classical SRS.

Keywords: relative precision, relative saving, order statistics, maximum likelihood estimator

1. Introduction

In public health related studies, the virus of measles is considered as highly epidemic and responsible for serious diseases. According to the medical dictionary, measles virus infects the lungs in children, which can cause pneumonia in older children, can cause inflammation of the brain, called encephalitis, which can cause seizures and brain damage [1]. As a preventive measure, adequate vaccination is introduced in early childhood to acquire immunity against measles virus. According to the Integrated Child Development Services Program (ICDS) in India, a child should have received the basic vaccines (BCG, polio, DPT and measles) at 12–23 months of age.

In this regard, the World Health Organization (WHO) launched the Expanded Program on Immunization (EPI) in May 1974 to immunize children around the world. Since then, it has been widely used to access coverage. India launched the National Vaccination Program entitled Expanded Programme of Immunization in 1978 with the introduction of the BCG, OPV, DPT and anti-typhoid-paratyphoid vaccine. The EPI was renamed and launched, with a major change in list of vaccinations, as the Universal Vaccination Program on 19 November 1985. The measles vaccine [2] has been added to latest schedule.

To study the vaccination coverage a few among various sampling procedures and are the most popular *viz.*, lot quality assurance sampling (LQAS) [3, 4], systematic sampling, cluster sampling [5] and stratified sampling [6], are based on simple random sampling (SRS) either at one stage or subsequent stage. In most of the practical situations to obtain actual measurement of an observation is not relatively easy and economical, but ranking a small subset of auxiliary information about a sample is relatively easy, economical and reliable. McIntyre in 1952 [7] have introduced the procedure of ranked set sampling (RSS), as an alternative, which is highly beneficial and much superior to the standard SRS, for estimating population parameters. In RSS procedure a set of units is randomly drawn from the population and the selected units are ranked by using judgment method or by other means which does not require actual measurement. Only the unit possessing lowest rank is measured for this set of units. Next, a second set of units of the same size is drawn as earlier and ranked; then the unit at the second lowest position is measured. This procedure of ranking and measuring is continued until we get as many observations as the size of the set. This entire procedure is regarded as a cycle. The process of cycle formation will be continued until the desired sample size is obtained for analysis.

Based on real-life primary data, in the present study, the procedure of RSS is investigated against SRS for estimating the proportion of children aged 12–23 months of slum and non-slum households of Guwahati, the capital city of state Assam, India, who are not immunized with the vaccine against measles. The information on a total of 500 (260 slum and 240 non-slum) households, were obtained after being ranked using mother's age 15–49 years (in months), as auxiliary variable is used as auxiliary variable. The data of the same size is obtained by following the SRS procedure, for the evaluation of the performance and effectiveness of the RSS estimator compared to SRS estimator.

2. Sampling design

The study population is a representative cross-sectional sample of children aged 12–23 months to mothers aged 15–49 of Guwahati City, India. Five hundred households, following both SRS and RSS procedures, having the children of age from 6 months to 5 years were identified for the present study. Following the SRS technique, from both slum and non-slum regions, a sample 250 households were obtained. Among the selected 500 households under RSS, 260 were residents of slum region whereas remaining 240 are of non-slum parts of the Guwahati City. The variable considered in the study is the proportion of children in Guwahati City, India who are not immunized with the vaccine against measles. It is assumed that the case of receiving the vaccination of children usually depends on the awareness of the child's mother on immunization. Lower the age of a mother who has children aged 12–23 months, lower would be the consciousness as expected. Therefore, the age of the mother (in months) was used as a ranking variable in RSS for classification of the sample. Information on children was obtained by a face to face interview with the mothers. Mothers were selected through RSS conducted in Guwahati City.

The observation were divided into m sets of size four ($s = 4$) each. The observations under RSS procedure are obtained through the following steps.

1. A simple random sample of units s^2 is selected from the target population and is distributed randomly in sets s, each with s units.

2. In each set s, the units are ranked according to the age of the mother. Since the samples in different sets are ranked according to the age of the mother (1, 2, 3, 4).

Obviously, there is a high chance of having ties then in this situation, the observations are ordered systematically in sequence, as explained by Terpstra and Nelson (2005).

3. From the first set, the unit corresponds to the mother with the lowest age (in months) is selected. From the second set, the unit corresponds to the mother with the second lowest age is selected and so on. Finally, from *sth* set, the unit corresponding to the mother with the highest age is selected. The other $s(s-1)$ sampled units are discarded from the data set.

4. Steps 1–3, called a cycle, are repeated m times to obtain a ranked set sample of size ms.

Corresponding to each selected mother, information regarding whether her child is administrated with measles vaccination or not is collected.

Suppose X is the binary response that takes value "1" if the child is vaccinated with measles vaccine and "0" otherwise. Let $\{X_{[i]j}, i = 1, 2, \cdots, s, j = 1, 2, \cdots, m\}$ represent a ranked set sample of size ms, where $X_{[i]j}$ takes the values "1" or "0" according as the jth child in the ith ranking class is vaccinated or not. By virtue of ranked set sampling all $X_{[i]j}'s$ are independently distributed. Here for any i from 1 to s, $X_{[i]1}, X_{[i]2}, \cdots, X_{[i]m}$ are independently and identically (i.i.d.) distributed. Here $X_{[i]1}$ can be regarded as the ith order statistic corresponding to a simple random sample of s observations, say, $(X_1, X_2, \cdots, X_s)$ on X. Obviously, X_is have the common probability mass function (p.m.f.) given by

$$f(x|p) = p^x(1-p)^{1-x}, \; x = 0, 1, \; 0 < p < 1, \tag{1}$$

where p is the probability that a child is vaccinated with measles vaccine in the population. Now we have, for any i, $1 \le i \le s$

$$P(X_{[i]1} = 1) = P(\text{among } X_{i'}s, \text{ at least } s - i + 1 \text{ X} - \text{values are } 1)$$

$$= \sum_{r=s-i+1}^{s} \binom{s}{i} p^r \, (1-p)^{s-r} = p_{[i]}, \text{ say,}$$

$$P(X_{[i]} = 0) = \left(1 - p_{[i]}\right).$$

Obviously, $p_{[i]}$ is the proportion, in ith class, of children who received the vaccination and p is the overall proportion of children receiving the vaccine in entire target population. Here it can be easily shown that

$$\sum_{r=1}^{s} p_{[r]} = sp. \tag{2}$$

3. Estimation of parameter p

For a dichotomous population, estimation of population proportion p, based on ranked set samples have already been investigated [8–14]. A method for estimation [15] of p using RSS for the situations where the binary variable is obtained from a continuous variable. Let $X_{RSS} = \left(\mathbf{X}_{[1]}, \cdots, \mathbf{X}_{[i]}, \cdots, \mathbf{X}_{[s]}\right)$, $\mathbf{X}_{[i]} = \left(X_{[i]1}, \cdots, X_{[i]m}\right)^T$ and $\mathbf{p} = \left(p_{[1]}\cdots, p_{[i]}, \cdots, p_{[s]}\right)$. Here $X_{[i]1}, \cdots, X_{[i]m}$ are i.i.d. Binomial $\left(1, p_{[i]}\right)$, $i = 1, 2, \cdots, s$. So the joint p.m.f. of $X_{[i]j}, j = 1, 2, \cdots, m$ is given by

$$f\left(\mathbf{x}_{[i]}|p_{[i]}\right) = \prod_{j=1}^{m} p_{[i]}^{x_{[i]j}}\left(1 - p_{[i]}\right)^{1-x_{[i]j}} = p_{[i]}^{z_i}\left(1 - p_{[i]}\right)^{m-z_i} \tag{3}$$

where $z_i = \sum_{i=1}^{m} x_{[i]j}$, the number of children getting vaccinated observed in ith ranking class of the given ranked set sample. Obviously, $Z_i = \sum_{i=1}^{m} X_{[i]j} \sim$ Binomial $\left(m, p_{[i]}\right)$, independently for all $i = 1, 2, \cdots, s$. Then the joint p.m.f. of the whole sample $\mathbf{X_{RSS}}$ is of the form

$$f(\mathbf{x_{RSS}}|\mathbf{p}) = \prod_{i=1}^{s} f\left(\mathbf{x}_{[i]}|p_{[i]}\right) = \prod_{i=1}^{s} p_{[i]}^{z_i}\left(1 - p_{[i]}\right)^{m-z_i}. \tag{4}$$

Applying standard maximum likelihood (ML) principle the ML estimate of p under ranked set sampling, is given by

$$\hat{p}_{RSS} = \underset{p}{arg\ \ max}\ f(\mathbf{x_{RSS}}|p).$$

Given the RSS data, the form of likelihood function of p is complicated and hence the MLE of p is difficult to obtain directly. Alternatively, for $i = 1, 2, \cdots, s$, one can separately derive ML estimate, say, $\hat{p}_{[i]}$ of based on the likelihood function (3) and then MLE of p can be formulated by using the relation (2) as

$$\hat{p}_{RSS} = \frac{1}{s}\sum_{i=1}^{s} \hat{p}_{[i]}.$$

Here, it can be shown that, for each $i = 1, 2, \cdots, s$, $\frac{Z_i}{m}$ would be the maximum likelihood estimator of $p_{[i]}$ and hence we get

$$\hat{p}_{RSS} = \frac{1}{s}\sum_{i=1}^{s} \frac{Z_i}{m} = \overline{X}_{RSS}, \ \text{say}, \tag{5}$$

where $\overline{X}_{RSS}$ is the overall mean of the ranked set sample.

Let $Y_1, Y_2, \cdots, Y_n$ are the observations drawn according to SRS design and $\hat{p}_{SRS}$ be an unbiased estimator of p, then the corresponding unbiased estimator of p can be obtained, as

$$\hat{p}_{SRS} = \sum_{i=1}^{n} \frac{y_i}{n} \tag{6}$$

4. Effect of imperfect ranking

The discussion done in the previous sections are based on the assumption that the ranking procedure produces the correct order statistics. But, a perfect ranking mechanism is very rare in practice and hence some error in judgment ranking is inevitable. So it is necessary to study how much robust the proposed procedure is against when the rankings are not perfect. Estimation of p under perfect and imperfect unbalanced RSS [13, 16, 17] are discussed.

Let $X_{[i]}$ and $X_{(i)}$ denote, respectively, the ith judgment order and i^{th} true order statistic while a set of s units are ordered. In the presence of ranking error, $X_{[i]}$ is not necessarily equal to $X_{(i)}$. Let π_{ij} denote the probability that the ith judgment order statistic actually have the true rank j, for $i = 1(1)s, j = 1(1)s$. Assume that π_{ij}s satisfy the conditions

$$0 \leq \pi_{ij} \leq 1, \quad \pi_{ij} = \pi_{ji}, \forall (i,j), \quad \sum_{j=1}^{s} \pi_{ij} = 1, \forall i, \quad \sum_{i=1}^{s} \pi_{ij} = 1, \forall j.$$

That is, $\boldsymbol{\pi} = \left(\pi_{ij}\right)$ is a doubly stochastic symmetric matrix of order $s \times s$. Under this assumption the distribution of $X_{[i]}$ would be changed to Binomial $(1, p^*_{[i]})$, for each $i = 1(1)s$, where

$$p^*_{[i]} = \sum_{j=1}^{s} \pi_{ij} p_{[j]}.$$

Equivalently,

$$\boldsymbol{p}^* = \boldsymbol{\pi} \boldsymbol{p}$$

where $\boldsymbol{p} = \left(p_{[1]}, p_{[2]}, \cdots, p_{[s]}\right)'$ and $\boldsymbol{p}^* = \left(p^*_{[1]}, p^*_{[2]}, \cdots, p^*_{[s]}\right)'$. For the present purpose we take the particular form of $\boldsymbol{\pi}$ as in [18, 19],

$$\boldsymbol{\pi} = \begin{pmatrix} \rho & \delta & \delta & \ldots & \delta \\ & \rho & \delta & \ldots & \delta \\ & & \rho & \ldots & \delta \\ & & & \ddots & \vdots \\ & & & & \rho \end{pmatrix}, \quad 0 < \rho < 1, \quad \delta = \frac{1-\rho}{s-1}.$$

Here "$\rho = 1$" corresponds to the case of perfect ranking. Under the above probability model for imperfect ranking some consequential facts are justified below.

1. $\sum_{i=1}^{s} p^*_{[i]} = sp$, that is, the present imperfect ranking mechanism is consistent

Justification:

$$\sum_{i=1}^{s} p^*_{[i]} = \sum_{i=1}^{s} \sum_{j=1}^{s} \pi_{ij} p_{[j]} = \sum_{j=1}^{s} \left(\sum_{i=1}^{s} \pi_{ij} \right) p_{[j]} = \sum_{j=1}^{s} p_{[j]} = sp$$

and hence

$$\sum_{i=1}^{s} \left(1 - p^*_{[i]}\right) = s(1-p),$$

so that

$$\frac{1}{s}\sum_{i=1}^{s} P\left(X_{[i]} = x\right) = P(X = x), \ \ for\ x = 0, 1.$$

2. For equal sample size, i.e., $n = ms$

$$Variance\left(\hat{p}_{RSS}\right) \leq Variance\left(\hat{p}_{SRS}\right)$$

Justification: For all $i = 1, 2, \cdots, s$, setting

$$a_i = \sum_{j=1}^{s} \pi_{ij} p_{[j]}, \quad b_i = \sum_{j=1}^{s} \pi_{ij}\left(1 - p_{[j]}\right),$$

one can get under ranked set sampling with the presence of ranking error

$$\begin{aligned} \text{Variance }(\hat{p}) &= \frac{1}{ms^2}\sum_{i=1}^{s} p^*_{[i]}\left(1 - p^*_{[i]}\right) \\ &= \frac{1}{ms^2}\sum_{i=1}^{s}\left(\sum_{j=1}^{s}\pi_{ij}p_{[j]}\right)\left(\sum_{j=1}^{s}\pi_{ij}\left(1 - p_{[j]}\right)\right) \\ &= \frac{1}{ns}\sum_{i=1}^{s} a_i b_i, \ \text{ say,} \end{aligned}$$

Also, for the above choice of $\boldsymbol{\pi}$-matrix, it is verified that

$$a_i = \delta s p + (\rho - \delta) p_{[i]} \ \text{ and } \ b_i = \delta s(1 - p) + (\rho - \delta)\left(1 - p_{[i]}\right). \tag{7}$$

Now, from the definition of $p_{[i]}$s, we argue that $\left\{p_{[i]}\right\}_{i=1(1)s}$ is a non-decreasing sequence and subsequently, among two sequences $\{a_i\}_{i=1(1)s}$ and $\{b_i\}_{i=1(1)s}$, one is non-decreasing and the other is non-increasing. So, from Chebyshev's inequality for a_is and b_is we have

$$\frac{1}{s}\sum_{i=1}^{s} a_i b_i \leq \left\{\frac{1}{s}\sum_{i=1}^{s} a_i\right\}\left\{\frac{1}{s}\sum_{i=1}^{s} b_i\right\}.$$

As we know that the variance of $\hat{p}$ in SRS is $\frac{p(1-p)}{n}$, the required justification follows from the fact that

$$\sum_{i=1}^{s} a_i = sp, \ \sum_{i=1}^{s} b_i = s(1 - p).$$

The justification in case of perfect ranking follows automatically by taking $\rho = 1$ in the above proof.

5. Comparison between $\hat{p}_{RSS}$ and $\hat{p}_{SRS}$

It is easy to argue that the ML estimates $\hat{p}_{[1]}, \hat{p}_{[2]}, \cdots, \hat{p}_{[s]}$ are statistically independent as the variables $Z_i's$ are independently distributed. Again, substituting the value $\frac{Z_i}{m}$ of $\hat{p}_{[i]}$ in Eq. (5), the estimate $\hat{p}_{RSS}$ can be shown to be identical with the overall mean of the given ranked set sample. It is also readily verified that $\hat{p}_{SRS}$ is an unbiased estimator of p.

The comparison of effectiveness and efficiency of the estimators based on simple random samples and ranked set samples, is obtained on the basis of criteria *viz.*, relative precision (RP) and relative saving (RS). The expressions for RP, RS and MSE of the estimators are described below as

$$RP = \frac{E(\hat{p}_{SRS} - p)^2}{E(\hat{p}_{RSS} - p)^2} = \frac{V(\hat{p}_{SRS})}{V(\hat{p}_{RSS})} \tag{8}$$

$$RS = \frac{V(\hat{p}_{SRS}) - V(\hat{p}_{RSS})}{V(\hat{p}_{SRS})}. \tag{9}$$

6. Result and discussion

Table 1 shows the estimates of proportion of measles immunized children in Assam, under SRS and RSS are very different but RSS based estimates 0.80 and 0.92 are very close to Census report for Assam (2012) [20] true value, which is 0.84 (rural) and 0.90 (urban), and has less variability than the SRS estimator and are very distinct from the true values. The estimate based on RSS is found to be 58% and 142%, for slum and non-slum region, respectively, more precision than that of SRS. Here, smaller the value of ρ represents higher will be the ranking error in RSS. The performance of estimates even in imperfect situation as compare to SRS, for different choices of the ranking error probability $\rho = 0.2, 0.6, 0.9$, shows the estimates based on RSS is 48%, 50% and 56% for slum region, and 139%, 140% and 141% for non-slum, respectively, more precision as compare to SRS. RSS also shows a saving of 37%(59%) under perfect and a minimum of 32%(58%) under imperfect in slum (non-slum) as compare to SRS.

Region	Criteria	*n*	SRS	*s*	*m*	RSS perfect	RSS imperfect		
							ρ =0.2	ρ =0.6	ρ =0.9
Slum	Estimate	250	0.64	4	65	0.80	0.80	0.80	0.80
	Variance		0.92			0.58	0.62	0.62	0.59
	RP					1.58	1.48	1.50	1.56
	RS					36.83	32.29	33.27	35.70
Non-slum	Estimate	250	0.74	4	60	0.92	0.92	0.92	0.92
	Variance		0.76			0.32	0.32	0.32	0.32
	RP					2.42	2.39	2.40	2.41
	RS					58.60	58.22	58.30	58.51

Table 1.
Estimate of proportion of immunized children (p), variance (in 10^{-3}), relative precision and relative saving (in %), in different regions of Guwahati under SRS, RSS perfect and imperfect procedures.

7. Conclusion

The present study revealed that RSS based estimates in both of perfect and imperfect situations, performs better than SRS based estimates. It should also be emphasized in context of estimation of proportion of measles immunization coverage in slum and non-slum region of Assam, RSS based estimates for different choices of accuracy (ρ) are not only more accurate but are more precise and efficient than the SRS procedure, and also suggest that the procedure of RSS is better than the classical SRS. Therefore, based on the obtained results one can recommend to adopt RSS procedure in epidemiological application and in other health related studies so that it will help in planning to build a healthy and disease free environment.

Acknowledgements

The first author would like to express his deepest gratitude and sincere thanks to the Department of Science & Technology, India (Grant No. IF130365) for funding. The second author acknowledges the financial support provided by Indian Council of Medical Research (ICMR), New Delhi (Grant No-69/40/2008 ECD-II). The authors would like to thank the anonymous referees and editorial board for their constructive comments and suggestions to improve the quality of this manuscript.

Author details

Vivek Verma[1*] and Dilip C. Nath[2]

1 Department of Neurology, All India Institute of Medical Sciences (AIIMS), New Delhi, India

2 Administration, Assam University, Silchar, Assam, India

*Address all correspondence to: viv_verma456@yahoo.com

References

[1] Orenstein WA, Perry RT, Halsey NA. The clinical significance of measles: A review. The Journal of Infectious Diseases. 2004;**189**(Suppl 1):S4-S16

[2] Lahariya C. A brief history of vaccines & vaccination in India. Indian Journal of Medical Research. 2014;**139**: 491-511

[3] Hoshaw-Woodard S. Description and Comparison of the Methods of Cluster Sampling and Lot Quality Assurance Sampling to Assess Immunization Coverage. Geneva: Department of Vaccines and Biologicals, World Health Organization; 2001

[4] Datta A, Mog C, Das S, Datta S. A cross-sectional study to assess the immunization coverage and vaccine dropout rates among 12 to 23 months old children in a rural area of Tripura. International Journal. 2017;**6**(2):394

[5] Singh J, Jain DC, Sharma RS, Verghese T. Evaluation of immunization coverage by lot quality assurance sampling compared with 30-cluster sampling in a primary health Centre in India. Bulletin of the World Health Organization. 1996;**74**(3):269

[6] Murhekar MV, Kamaraj P, Kanagasabai K, Elavarasu G, Rajasekar TD, Boopathi K, et al. Coverage of childhood vaccination among children aged 12–23 months, Tamil Nadu, 2015, India. Indian Journal of Medical Research. 2017;**145**(3):377

[7] McIntyre GA. A method for unbiased selective sampling, using ranked sets. Australian Journal of Agricultural Research. 1952;**3**(4):385-390

[8] Terpstra JT, Miller ZA. Exact inference for a population proportion based on a ranked set sample. Communications in Statistics-Simulation and Computation. 2006; **35**(1):19-26

[9] Kvam PH. Ranked set sampling based on binary water quality data with covariates. Journal of Agricultural, Biological, and Environmental Statistics. 2003;**8**(3):271-279

[10] Chen H. Alternative ranked set sample estimators for the variance of a sample proportion. Applied Statistics Research Progress. 2008;**35**

[11] Chen H, Stasny EA, Wolfe DA. Ranked set sampling for efficient estimation of a population proportion. Statistics in Medicine. 2005;**24**(21): 3319-3329

[12] Chen H, Stasny EA, Wolfe DA. Improved procedures for estimation of disease prevalence using ranked set sampling. Biometrical Journal. 2007; **49**(4):530-538

[13] Chen H, Stasny AE, Wolfe AD, MacEachern NS. Unbalanced ranked set sampling for estimating a population proportion under imperfect rankings. Communications in Statistics: Theory and Methods. 2009;**38**(12):2116-2125

[14] Verma V, Nath CD, Das R. Bayesian bounds for population proportion under ranked set sampling. Communications in Statistics-Simulation and Computation. 2019;**48**(2):478-493

[15] Verma V, Das R, Nath CD. Bayesian Cramer-Rao lower bound of variances under ranked set sampling. Materials Today Proceedings. 2018;**5**(1): 1747-1758

[16] Lacayo H, Neerchal NK, Sinha BK. Ranked set sampling from a dichotomous population. Journal of Applied Statistical Science. 2002;**11**(1): 83-90

[17] Chen H, Stasny EA, Wolfe DA. Unbalanced ranked set sampling for estimating a population proportion. Biometrics. 2006;**62**(1):150-158

[18] Terpstra JT, Nelson EJ. Optimal rank set sampling estimates for a population proportion. Journal of Statistical Planning and Inference. 2005; **127**(1):309-321

[19] Hatefi A, Jozani MJ. Fisher information in different types of perfect and imperfect ranked set samples from finite mixture models. Journal of Multivariate Analysis. 2013;**119**:16-31

[20] Registrar General of India. Annual Health Survey 2011-12 FACT SHEET Assam. New Delhi: Ministry of Health and Family Welfare, Department of Family Welfare; 2012. Available at: http://www.censusindia.gov.in/vital_statistics/AHSBulletins/AHS_Factsheets_2011_12/Assam _Factsheet_2011–12.pdf

Chapter 10

A Role for the Measles Virus in Oncology

Daniel Benharroch

Abstract

An association between the measles virus (MV) and classic Hodgkin lymphoma (CHL) was reported by our center in Beer-Sheva, starting in 2003. Our basic evidence on the relationship had been established by immunohistochemistry, using several commercial and specific experimental anti-measles antibodies in about 50% of our patients. It relied also on the reverse transcriptase-polymerase chain reaction (RT-PCR) and *in situ* hybridization (ISH) of MV RNA, and overall, was essentially descriptive. The first and only response to our thesis was advanced in 2007 in doublet articles, in a single issue of a Cancer Journal. Our conclusions were hereby dismissed. Since reservations relating the above refutation seemed self-evident, the subsequent publication of several of our articles was launched. They disclosed evidence of an association of the MV with further categories of cancers, as well as its absence in some distinct tumors. A mechanism by which the MV may regulate apoptosis in the tumor cells of CHL was also proposed. A suspected role for the MV in oncomodulation is advocated. We deplore, however, the absence of further interest in our hypothesis among world experts.

Keywords: classic Hodgkin lymphoma, measles virus, antigens, RT-PCR, in situ hybridization, endometrial carcinoma, breast cancer, lung cancer

1. Introduction

Classic Hodgkin lymphoma (CHL) stands out among malignant tumors, by the relative paucity of the tumor cells in the involved lymph nodes. These Hodgkin and Reed-Sternberg (H/RS) cells (**Figure 1**) are distributed unevenly within the majority of inflammatory cells, fibrosis and necrosis [1]. It is understood that, independent of the proportion of H/RS cells in CHL, the outcome of the malignancy will be favorable, with a cure rate of 75–90% [2, 3]. Such a therapeutic success is unusual for cancer at large.

When considering the many prognostics and risk factors regarding CHL, the stage of the tumor, as expected, is the most relevant. Evidence of systemic symptoms: fever higher than 38°C for at least a month; weight loss of more than 10% of body weight, lasting 6 months or more, and/or drenching night sweats, singly or collectively, worsen the prognosis [1]. A difference is described between genders, as females fare as a rule better than males, no consideration being given to a higher incidence of nodular sclerosis CHL in females. Indeed, children and older adult males with mixed cellularity CHL, especially in developing countries, get on worse with the disease [2, 4]. In contrast, females would be included in the bulk of CHL patients, aged 15–36, with a favorable outcome [5].

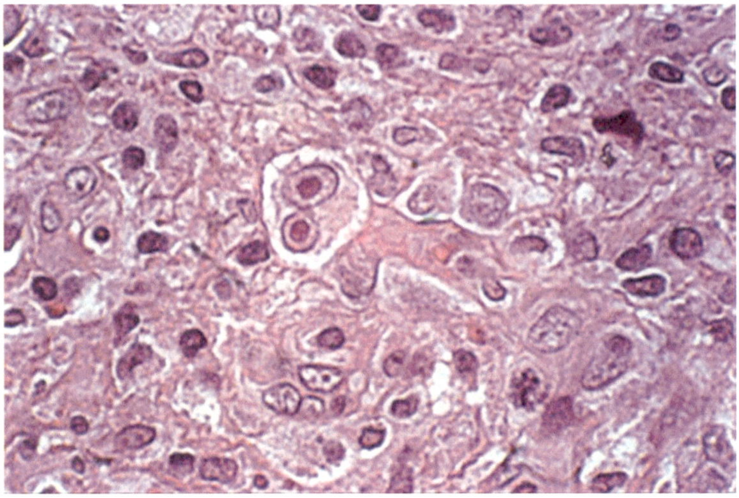

Figure 1.
Section of lymph node from a patient with classic HL. Off center is a Hodgkin/Reed-Sternberg giant tumor cell (H&E × 360).

Some 15-20% of human cancers are thought to arise by mechanisms which concern viruses, bacteria, or parasites [6, 7]. Evidence for their involvement comes partly from the detection of the microorganism in biopsies and partly from epidemiological and animal studies. Viruses might modify cellular genes directly, as with RNA tumor viruses, or may affect cell proliferation, as with DNA tumor viruses, and thus contribute to neoplasm formation [6, 7]. As a rule, the virus is responsible for only a limited number of steps in the promotion or progression of cancer. In most cases, the precise role of cancer-associated virus is hard to decipher, due to the long delay from the initial viral infection [6]. In any case, the number of human beings infected with the above viruses is much larger by far from that of patients who develop cancer. Therefore, tumor viruses probably act in conjunction with additional factors [7].

Chronic inflammation may play an important role in the above processes as well as in other pathologic events which may lead to cancer [8]. In some cases of unresolved chronic inflammation, the immune response becomes maladaptive, hence promoting tumorigenesis [8]. A regenerative process supported by an array of bioactive mediators, promote cell survival, tissue remodeling, and angiogenesis. The mediators will also cause genomic stress and mutations [9].

A correlation between CHL and the Epstein-Barr virus (EBV) has been demonstrated many years ago [10, 11], with a causal relationship being established as soon as 2001 [12]. The incidence of EBV infection in CHL has shown a wide geographic variation, from 17 to 30% in industrialized countries, to as high as 100% in some developing countries [13, 14]. Several more years elapsed before the distribution of EBV infection by gender, age, and CHL type was determined (**Figure 2**) [13, 14]. Thus, EBV is expressed more frequently in males, notably in children from developing countries, as well as in older adults all over the globe, these two groups showing as a rule mixed cellularity CHL. Female CHL patients stand out, in general, by showing nodular sclerosis CHL with a markedly lower level of EBV expression and a young adult age (15–36) [15]. A small subset of young adult males will develop CHL after recovering from infectious mononucleosis [16]. The EBV is recognized as oncogenic. Specifically, its transforming potential, with cell proliferation, inflammation, and apoptosis arrest, has been related to the nuclear factor-κB (NF-κB) and the EBV/LMP1 will further contribute to the inhibition of the H/RS cell apoptosis [15–19]. As noted, EBV does not play a significant role in the largest subset of CHL that affect young adults and most of the female CHL patients.

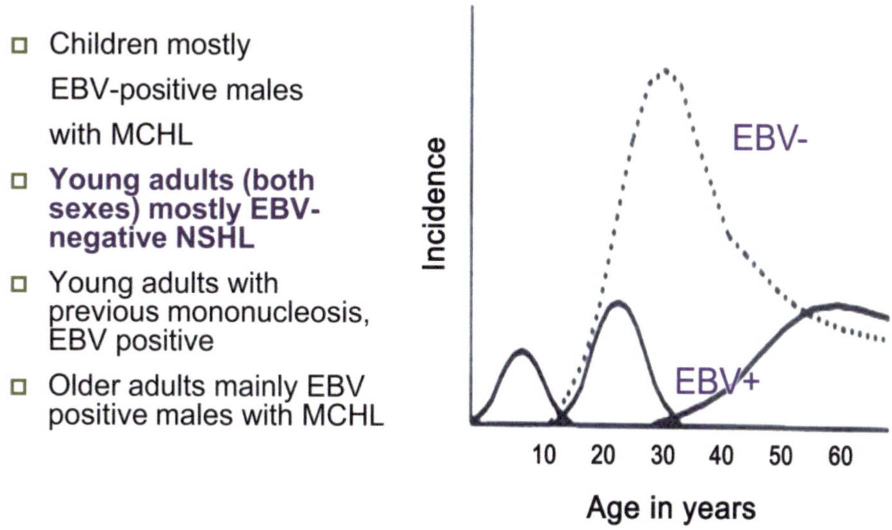

Figure 2.
Association between age, gender, EBV expression, and classic Hodgkin lymphoma, including the types thereof.

The above subset of young adult female patients corresponds to that defined in the hallmark epidemiological studies in the early 1980s as patients with the "late host response model" [15–19]. These patients are considered to be submitted to the late exposure to a common infectious agent, the term "late" meaning that instead of coming across the common infectious agent for the first time in early childhood, this occurs at adolescence or young adulthood. The epidemiological thesis further suggests that these individuals had a late encounter with the agent, since they had few and late contacts with other children (single child, individual family house, and child who skipped the kindergarten) [15]. To account for the late host response model, it is suggested that a common agent, probably a virus, reaches the organism for the first time at a stage in which the metabolism and/or the hormonal balance is markedly different from that of a toddler, the age at which the encounter regularly takes place. At this point, the internal environment has varied deeply and probably, so has the immune system [15–19]. Thus, it seems that the EBV plays a relatively minor role, in the largest subset of the CHL that is most prevalent in industrialized countries [18].

When looking for a substitute for the EBV in CHL, it was observed that none of the additional viruses, HHV-6, -7, -8, polyoma JC virus, SV40, HTLV-1 and -2, and human retrovirus 5, once considered as possible candidates, have been detected in CHL tissues [20–26]. The only virus to be incompletely excluded at that time was the HCMV. However, one distinct virus showed qualities and associations which recalled to various extents of those of CHL.

The "candidate" proposed by us is the measles virus (MV). It penetrates the organism through the oropharynx. But, since it is lymphotropic, it enters the adjacent lymphoid tissues. This may account for the vast majority of CHL starting in cervical and/or in mediastinal lymph nodes [12, 27]. Histologically, it elaborates multinucleated cells—the Warthin-Finkeldey polykaryons. Of note, these polykaryons differ largely from the H/RS cells of CHL, mainly by the number of nuclei (up to 70) as well as by their phenotype (they are T-lymphocytes) [28]. An acute measles infection is soon followed, on the one hand by a life-long specific immunity, but also, paradoxically a transient cellular immune deficiency systematically develops. This deficiency lasts about 6 months, but at times, may last longer. The cellular immune deficiency which affects CHL patients is not different in principle, but it may be long lasting [12].

At the time our thesis was formulated, the type of MV neural infection known as subacute sclerosing panencephalitis (SSPE) was considered one of the very few persistent MV infections, most being CNS slow viral infections. However, it was difficult to grasp a possible association between MV and cancer, which would not account for the long lapse of time necessary for the malignant transformation. In that context, the absence of a persistent MV infection might be counterproductive. The alternative being that against all odds, MV may be oncogenic, and the MV is not among the consensually recognized oncogenic viruses! An additional clue to MV causing a persistent infection beyond the CNS is the absence of membrane expression of hemagglutinin MV antigens, although this lack of expression might be due also to the lymph node mode of fixation [29].

2. Materials and methods

The basic part of our study (2003–2004) concerned 154 patients with CHL diagnosed between 1975 and 2000 at the Soroka University Medical Centre in Beer-Sheva, Israel, whose tissues were available for research. Only pretreatment biopsies with confirmed histological type, by two hematopathologists were included. Clinical data were retrieved from the patients' charts and when those were not found, the details were searched in the Israel Population Registry by linkage.

2.1 Immunohistochemistry

Immunophenotyping was performed on formalin-fixed, paraffin-embedded (FFPE) tissues by the avidin-biotin peroxidase complex method and the Vectastain kit by Vector Laboratories (Burlingame, CA, USA) as described. The EBV/LMP1 antibody was purchased from Dako (Glostrup, Denmark); the anti-MV antibodies were either commercial: anti-nucleoprotein (NP)-MV; anti-hemagglutinin (HA)-MV; anti-matrix (M)-MV; and anti-phosphoprotein (P)-MV were purchased from Chemicon International Inc. (Temecula, CA, USA). Further experimental antibodies were a gift from Birrer et al. [30]: anti-NP, H14; and from Schneider-Schaulies et al. [31]: anti-NP, L39/22; L39/61 or anti-HA antibodies, K83; L77. The antibody specificity had been demonstrated by Western blotting. The staining was considered positive if 10% of H/RS cells or more were positive. For stringency purposes, we requested positivity for two MV antigens, for a case to be considered positive. A murine neuroblastoma cell line permanently infected by MV was used as a positive control; the same cell line, but non-infected was used as a negative control. These cell lines were also the controls used for the RT-PCR and ISH assays. Twenty-five cases of non-Hodgkin lymphoma were also tested by IHC.

2.2 Reverse transcriptase-polymerase chain reaction

Total RNA was obtained by extraction of snap-frozen lymph node samples from part of our patients, when available. For this goal, EZ-RNA Total RNA Isolation Kit (Biological Industries Co., Beit Ha-Emek, Israel) was employed, using the manufacturer's instructions. To each sample, 40 U of RNA-guard (Promega, Madison, WI, USA) were added. One step RT-PCR was performed with Ready To Go ™ RT-PCR beads (Amersham Pharmacia Biotech Europe GbmH, Freiburg, Germany). A measure of 3 μl of RNA (2-6 μg) was used for each reaction. For the primers used in this study, see Table 1 from Ref. [3]. Nested PCR was carried out, using SUPER-NOVA DNA polymerase (Roche Molecular Biochemicals, Mannheim, Germany).

Total RNA was also retrieved from several FFPE tissues from CHL patients, using the Paraffin Block RNA Isolation Kit (Ambion Inc., The RNA Company, Austin, TX. USA) and RT-PCR followed by nested PCR carried out with 10 μl RNA, as described above. As controls, we used seven cases of non-Hodgkin lymphomas, one CHL which was negative for MV by IHC. As housekeeping genes, we used β-actin and protein phosphatase 2C β (pp2Cβ) considered appropriate for experiments related with low amounts of RNA.

To confirm our RT-PCR findings, the cDNA products of the nested PCR were blotted to GeneScreen (NEN Research Products, Boston, MA, USA) and hybridized to either an NP-MV probe (*CAATCCCTGGAGATTCCTCA*) or to a HA-MV probe (*GCTGGAAGCTGACACCTTTC*), labeled [γ-^{32} P] ATP (Amersham).

2.3 *In situ* hybridization on paraffin sections

The digoxigenin (DIG)-labeled antisense and sense probes to MV-specific mRNAs were prepared by linearizing the plasmids containing NP-MV including positions 105–586, and those including HA-MV encompassing positions 8147–8482 in PGEM-T Easy Vectors (Promega), with *Sal*I or *Sac*II. *In vitro* transcription was performed with the DIG-RNA Labeling kit, with SP6 for NP antisense and HA sense probes and T7 for NP sense and HA antisense DIG-labeled probes. The quality of the probes was determined by dot blotting, using a DIG-DNA detection kit (Roche Molecular Biochemicals), according to the manufacturer instructions, with minor modifications. *In situ* hybridization was performed, using Ogata's technique with certain modifications [32]. Paraffin sections were deparaffinized, rehydrated, and submitted to microwave in the presence of 10 mM MgCl2 buffer (pH 6) for 5 min at 750 W. Sections were allowed to cool down for 20 min and then digested with 20 μg/ml proteinase K for 10 min at 37°C. They were then fixed in paraformaldehyde in 0.1 M phosphate buffer containing 50% formamide, 10 mM Tris-HCl (pH 7.6), 200 μg/ml tRNA, 1 x Denhardt's solution, 10% dextran sulphate, 600 mM NaCl, 0.25% SDS, and 1 mM EDTA, pH 8.0. Hybridized DIG-labeled probes were detected by the DIG-Nucleic Acid Detection kit (Roche Molecular Biochemicals), followed by blocking with 1.5% of the blocking reagent included in the kit. The color reaction was stopped with 10 mM Tris-HCl (pH 7.6) and 1 mM EDTA. Sections were then fixed in 4% paraformaldehyde in phosphate-buffered saline and stained with hematoxylin. In addition to the neuroblastoma cell lines used as positive and negative controls, CHL cases negative for MV by IHC and NHL served as controls.

2.4 Comparison between IHC, RT-PCR, and ISH

This was performed on a sampling of cases. For this purpose, IHC positivity to a single NP-MV or HA-MV antibody was considered sufficient.

2.5 Clinicopathological correlations

Emphasis was given to MV IHC and to EBV-LMP1 expression, as RT-PCR and ISH disclosed much less results. For contingency table analysis, the $\chi 2$ or Fisher's exact test was used as appropriate.

3. Preliminary results

The lymph node tissues of 82 of 154 CHL patients were positive for at least two MV antigens (**Figure 3**). Neutralization of immunostaining was made possible by incubation of the primary anti-NP-MV antibody with the corresponding NP-MV peptide (**Figure 3b**). This assay confirms the specificity of the anti-NP-MV antibody in this context. Twenty-five cases of non-Hodgkin lymphoma (NHL) were totally negative for MV antigens.

A Southern blotting of the nested PCR shows several bands, some stronger, others faint, disclosing more hemagglutinin (HA, H) MV positivity, as compared with NP-MV positivity (**Figure 4**). Samples from 7 NHL were negative. Thus, in our laboratory, HA-MV RNA was positive in 4 of 15 cases, while only 2 of 16 NP-MV RNAs were expressed by the Southern blot in CHL.

Upon sequencing and alignment of three of the experiment products, we displayed an almost complete homology with the control (see [3] for details on the homology).

In situ hybridization on paraffin sections shows a strong cytoplasmic staining in the positive control (persistently MV infected murine neuroblastoma cell line) (upper left). The same cell line uninfected by MV was negative. An H/RS cell shows strong cytoplasmic positivity with NP-MV (lower left). Positive granular staining of several H/RS cells is disclosed in the right lower quadrant (**Figure 5**). Altogether, 2 of 7 CHL sections submitted for ISH were positive for HA-MV RNAs, while 8 of 21 were positive for NP-MV RNAs.

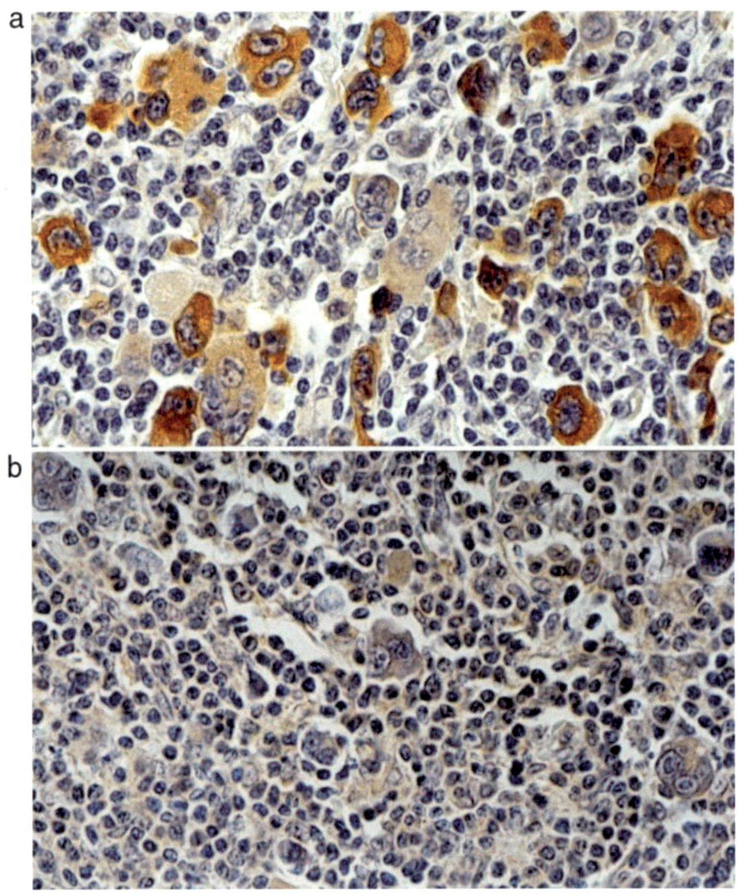

Figure 3.
Classic Hodgkin lymphoma-nucleoprotein-MV expression. a. Positive cytoplasmic immunostain of Hodgkin/Reed-Sternberg cells. b. Immunostaining following neutralization of antibody with a relevant MV peptide (Immunoperoxidase with DAB × 320).

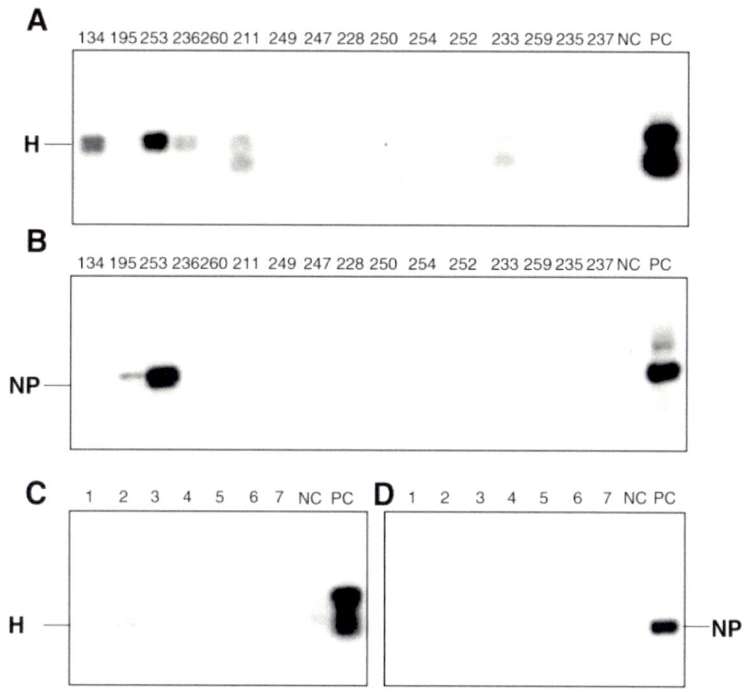

Figure 4.
Southern blotting based on cDNA from RT-PCR: A. A few cases of CHL show bands positive for hemagglutinin-MV (PC—positive control). B. Isolated bands, positive for nucleoprotein-MV. C and D. Absence of expression of MV in non-Hodgkin lymphomas.

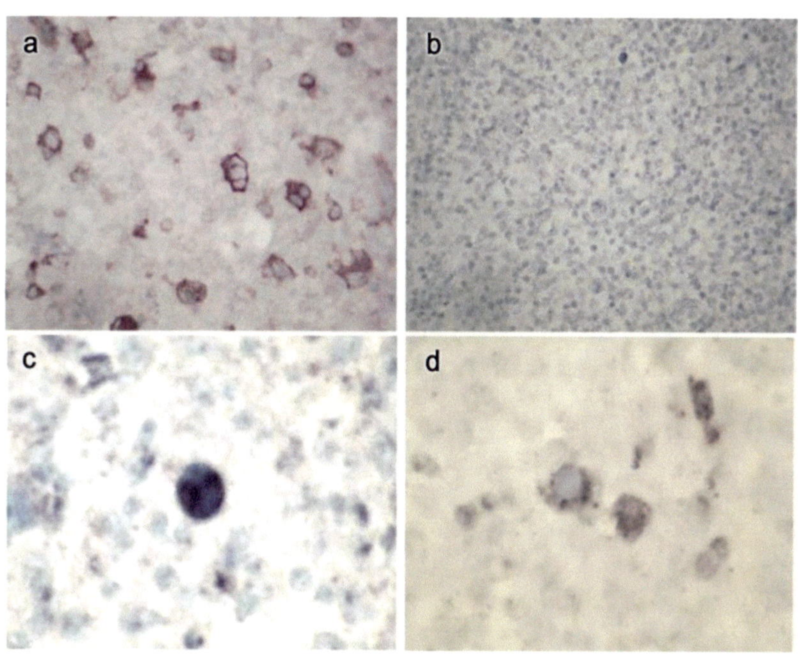

Figure 5.
In situ hybridization with MV-RNA. a. Positive control, using a murine, MV-transfected cell line. b. Negative control, with a non-transfected cell line. c. A Hodgkin/Reed-Sternberg cell disclosing positive cytoplasm for MV-NP-RNA. d. H/RS cells showing a granular cytoplasmic positivity for MV-HA-RNA.

A clinicopathological correlation was based on the immunophenotypic findings, as the specificity of the antibodies had been sustained by Western blotting and since, in each case, the immunostain had been confirmed with more than two antibodies. Last, the immunohistochemical (IHC) study had released the most manageable results.

Table 1 shows a statistically significant expression of MV antigens in female patients, in nodular sclerosis (NS) CHL, as compared with mixed cellularity (MC) CHL. A significant correlation was exhibited between negative CD15 and p53, and the negative expression of MV. **Table 2** displays a statistically significant expression of MV antigens compounded by the expression of EBV/LMP1, in NS-CHL, significantly more than that in MC-CHL, in early clinical stages, with apoptotic index lower than median and with the positive expression of MDM2.

A multivariable logistic regression model of the association of prognostic factors with dying from CHL, in 89 patients, is shown. Stage IV, as compared with the remainder, carried a significantly poorer prognosis, thus confirming that our cohort was representative. The compound expression of MV and EBV, specifically of MV+; EBV−, as well as MV−; EBV− was displayed as poor risk factors in our patients (**Table 3**).

		MV+	MV−	*p* Value
		n (%)	n (%)	
Total		82 (54.3)	69 (45.7)	
Gender	F	40 (**64.5**)	28 (35.5)	0.036
	M	42 (47.2)	47 (52.8)	
Subtype	NS	58 (**68.2**)	27 (31.8)	0.0013
	MC	21 (40.4)	31 (59.6)	
CD15	pos	77 (59.7)	52 (40.3)	0.015
	neg	4 (26.7)	11 (**73.3**)	
p53	pos	72 (61.5)	45 (38.5)	0.017
	neg	5 (31.3)	11 (**68.8**)	

Table 1.
Associations of classic Hodgkin lymphoma with the measles virus.

		MV+; LMP−	MV−; LMP+	*p* Value
Subtype	NS	45 (**86.5**)	7 (13.5)	0.00008
	MC	11 (44)	14 (56)	
Stage	I–IIA	22 (**84.6**)	4 (15.4)	0.023
	IIB–IVB	22 (57.9)	16 (42.1)	
BCL-2	Pos.	31 (**93.9**)	2 (6.1)	0.0001
	Neg.	27 (54)	23 (46)	
MDM-2	Pos.	36 (**87.8**)	5 (12.2)	0.0013
	Neg.	18 (54.5)	15 (45.5)	
Apop index	<Median	31 (**81.6**)	7 (18.4)	0.024
	>Median	22 (42.1)	16 (57.9)	

Table 2.
Hodgkin lymphoma—association with measles and Epstein-Barr viruses.

Factor	Odds ratio	95% CI	*p* Value
Gender	1.32	0.34–5.18	0.69
Stage	**13.67**	2.3–80.5	0.004
Bcl-2	0.34	0.08–1.44	0.34
MV+; EBV−	**10.05**	0.98–103.47	0.05
MV−; EBV+	1.53	0.07–35.44	0.79
MV−; EBV−	**15.2**	1.05–220.3	0.04

Table 3.
Multivariable logistic regression model of association of prognostic factors with dying of HL in 89 patients.

4. Interim discussion

The results of the first part of our study (2004) are summarized [3]. The association between MV and CHL, in a descriptive investigation, does not contain, so far, causal elements. This linkage is sustained by older epidemiologic studies describing brain and spinal cord tumors, as well as CHL, which followed exposure to the MV around the time of birth [33, 34]. They also suggest sporadic cases of CHL regression, occurring after acute measles infection or an MV vaccine [35–38]. Moreover, viral childhood infections, including measles, have been reported to protect from CHL occurrence [39].

Early clinical correlations exhibit more females, more NS-CHL, and more early stage cases, among patients with positive MV expression in their lymph node tissues. Nevertheless, positive MV expression in CHL seems to be related with a worse prognosis. One cannot refute the loss of the advantage conferred to the above variables by an MV infection, as expressed in the H/RS cells of CHL. Any mechanism involving the MV in CHL, if uncovered, should correlate with a worse outcome of the malignancy.

5. The refutation episode

Two years following the publication of the above-mentioned article and several months after the presentation of a poster at the Hodgkin Lymphoma Meeting in Kiel, a scientist, from Germany, contacted me indirectly, informing me that he wanted to investigate our findings. He proposed to find out whether he could reproduce our data in his lab. He also requested to make any fresh-frozen CHL tissues available to him, mainly those which showed an MV-antigen positivity.

In their labs, the German scientists had collected 44 frozen CHL samples, of which, only 18 were selected for their high quality RNA, as determined by the Agilent technology, as well as for classic H/RS cell morphology. Using UV-laser beam single cell microdissection, some 100 H/RS cells were pooled for each experiment. Total RNA was extracted and RT-PCR was performed with primers from three MV genes, which were different from those we had used in Israel [40].

Five CHL-derived cell lines were found to be negative for the three MV transcripts. Moreover, the 18 selected German cases did not show, either, evidence of any of the three viral transcripts. The GAPDH gene, used as a housekeeper gene for these experiments, displayed a large amount of RNA. At this point, the German group had received the 22 snap-frozen CHL samples from our laboratory. The cases had been chosen, as requested for their positive MV antigens, as shown on FFPE tissues. However, the selection highlighted only 7 of these cases, chosen for the high RNA quality and the classic H/RS cell features [40].

	NP-MV		HA-MV	
	Positive/n	(%)	Positive/n	(%)
RT-PCR	1/16	(6.25)	7/21	(33.3)
ISH	7/14	(50)	4/7	(57.1)
IHC	25/29	(86.2)	20/29	(68.9)

NP, nucleoprotein; HA, hemagglutinin; MV, measles virus; RT-PCR, reverse transcriptase-polymerase chain reaction; ISH, in situ hybridization; and IHC, immunohistochemistry.

Table 4.
Comparison of results obtained by three assays.

All 25 RNA samples disclosed negative results with the three MV transcripts, as studied in Essen labs. Back to Israel, 5 of 12 German histological unstained slides, subjected to IHC, were found to express MV antigens in the H/RS cells. A similar discrepancy in favor of IHC was also obtained in our series (**Table 4**).

The German scientists invited one of my colleagues and myself to co-author their manuscript. At every stage, we were reluctant to accept the invitation, due to the concern for a permanent damage to our hypothesis. Moreover, we did not curb our criticism, which covered several aspects of the manuscript. Prominent among these was the tight selection of the cases (both those from Germany and Israel). The methods used in Essen differed markedly from ours, notably the single cell micro-dissection, a different strategy for the RT-PCR and the choice of primers. Following our criticism, minor changes were introduced, but the German group did not go all the way: "....due to their worry that the manuscript will lose its sharp edge and might not be accepted by a highly rated journal."

The Scott collaborators of the Essen scientists reported above selected a group of patients, many of whom having suffered from measles, mainly as children. We consider this selection as counterproductive, since these patients should have been protected from the development of CHL. The very fact that they were not refutes the prevalent thesis that exposure of a child, aged 1–4 years, to MV infection protects the subject from CHL at a young-adult age [41]. The Scottish group may have had their own agenda, which might have unsettled the question raised by us. In addition, the antibody used by the Scott group is problematic: the clone 49–41 was purchased by us from Argene-Biosoft, Varilhes, France (# 11-045). It was not an anti-nucleoprotein antibody, as stated, and was positive in our lab for 37 of our 72 CHL cases (data not shown). Moreover, not unlike the German scientists, the Scotts used the GAPDH gene as a housekeeping gene, and we have already mentioned why it was not appropriate.

I have to admit, that we not only considered ourselves as the minor partner, but that we were such indeed! We had been recurrently reassured by the German scientists and by then had our two names included in the manuscript as co-authors. However, when we read the finalized doublet articles (in addition, the article by Wilson et al., weighted heavily on the balance) [41], published in the International Journal of Cancer, we realized that we had made a huge mistake.

The days which followed the double publication were crucial, since we were not sure, as co-authors, whether we were entitled to carry out an "insider" censure. When we read the final paper, we grasped the experience in terms of a possible deception. In addition to the impediments mentioned above, we also noted that the housekeeping gene, the GAPDH, might not be an adequate choice at all, since we had shown that CHL is most probably of low MV-RNA abundance. In contrast, the Essen group had described in relation with GAPDH a large amount of RNA [40]. Moreover, of the seven Israeli cases, selected for the experiment in Germany, five had been shown by us to present a faint MV-RNA positivity only (two) or were negative (three).

An independent putative evidence for a role of the MV in carcinogenesis is that part of the MV proteins that interacts with and stabilizes the Pirh2 protein, an ubiquitin E3 ligase, by preventing its ubiquitination. Pirh2 indeed negatively regulates p53 by targeting it for degradation in the proteasome.

Altogether, our criticism of the article, in which we took officially a part, is in principle that the German scientists carried out an investigation, which was by their declared intention, a duplication of our own research [3]. However, their study was anything, except a duplicate of ours! It stands out independently, with major flaws, notably a very strong selection of cases, the use of questionable primers of a housekeeping gene which is not appropriate for the expected amount of retrieved MV-RNA. It is of note that when confronted with our criticism regarding the manuscript, the German group seemed to agree, but did not modify the manuscript: "...for fear of weakening our data". Moreover, they insisted on mentioning the relevance of the findings to the CHL pathogenesis, which was not appropriate at this stage nor was it agreed upon [40]!

At this point, we insist that the impact of the European group refutation, on a possible role of MV in CHL, was extremely ruinous to our position and thesis. Moreover, its repercussions are felt to this day: for the reasons mentioned above, not a single investigator has accepted to engage in this project anymore, together with us or independently. By so doing, the two research groups have categorically "buried" our hypothesis. At the same time, we felt a release from the constraints which might have led us freeze in our position and we allowed ourselves again to indulge in the research concerning the measles virus and cancer. Therefore, we first wrote a review on our experience, as described above [42, 43].

6. New evidence

We set out to delve into endometrial carcinoma (EC), looking for the footprints of the MV in this cancer. Our cohort of EC included 49 patients, 36 of whom had a known follow-up. Using IHC and several anti-MV antibodies, we disclosed that 26 of the 36 (72%) did express MV antigens in tumor cells, mainly in type I EC (**Figure 6**). In addition, 16/21 of the patients displayed positivity for MV-RNA by ISH. When type II EC was allied with MV, then deeper myometrial invasion and a higher mortality were evident [44].

Our next endeavor concerned the possible role of MV in lung cancer. Our interest was first raised by the probable relevance of Pirh2 in lung cancer. Indeed, Pirh2, an E3 ubiquitin ligase, was found to be expressed in lung cancer, in which it inhibits p53 [45]. It was later found that the P-protein of the MV inhibited the function of Pirh2 (see description in [48]). This indirect association between lung cancer, Pirh2 and p53, and MV led us to the following study. We identified 65 non-small cell lung cancers, for which FFPE tissues were available over 10 years. We limited our study to the IHC analysis with several anti-MV antibodies (**Figure 7**). Of the cases included, 54/65 were positive for MV antigens. These 54 positive cases were associated with older patient age, with positive Pirh2 expression, as well as with an improved survival [46].

The following study concerned breast cancer and the MV-IHC expression. We identified 131 breast cancer cases, with preserved FFPE tissues. Of these cases, 64% were positive for the MV antigens (**Figure 8**). Positive MV expression was associated with ER ($p = 0.018$); with Ki-67 < 40% ($p = 0.029$); with low or intermediate grade ($p = 0.037$); with age < 50 ($p = 0.039$); and with p53 overexpression ($p = 0.049$) (**Table 5**). It seems, therefore, that the MV may play a role in the development of this cancer [47].

We have speculated whether the MV phosphoprotein, through its relation with the Pirh2, ubiquitin ligase, by itself negatively related with the p53 expression, may have more relevance, *a priori,* than other MV antigens to the pathogenesis of the

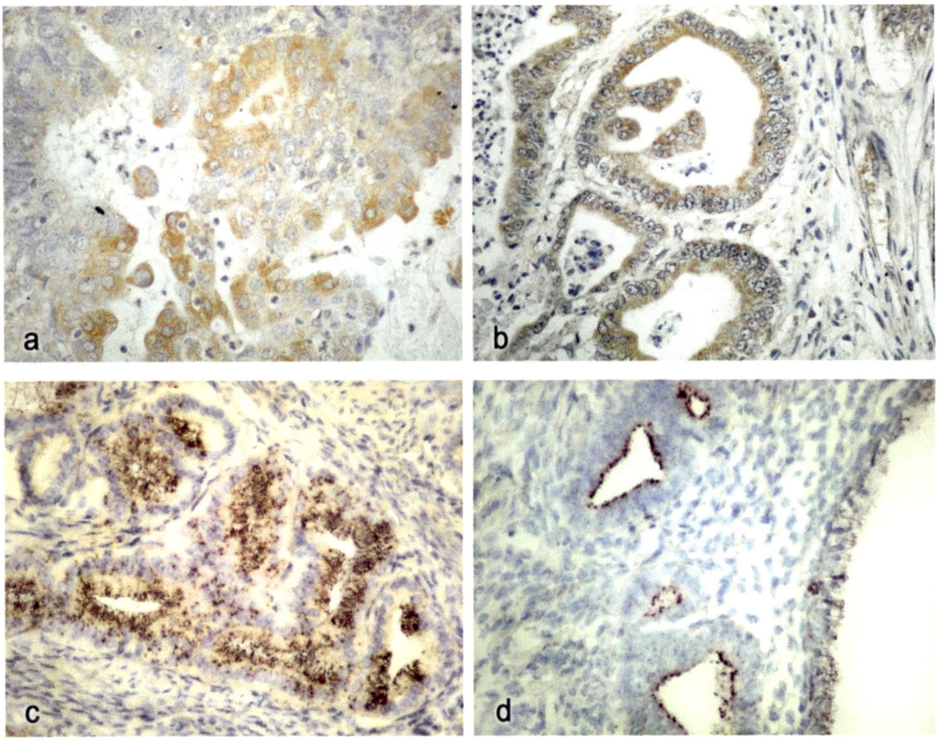

Figure 6.
Endometrial carcinoma—MV expression in tumor cells and in normal endometrium. a. Cytoplasmic HA-MV antigen is positive. b. Positive immunostain for NP-MV antigen. c. ISH positivity for NP-MV in tumoral glands. d. ISH positivity of surface and glandular normal epithelium of the case shown in c.

MV-associated cancer [48]. We therefore purchased a robust anti-MV-phosphoprotein antibody (9H4): sc-101,356, Santa Cruz Biotechnology, and used it by Western blot, first, to determine whether we could find a variance between the different types of lung cancers and in addition to determine whether the normal lung tissues around the tumor did express the MV. But, the distribution of lung cancer types in our cohort was clearly in favor of adenocarcinoma, which expressed the P-MV in 11 patients (84.6%). This was also the rate of its expression in the normal lung tissue

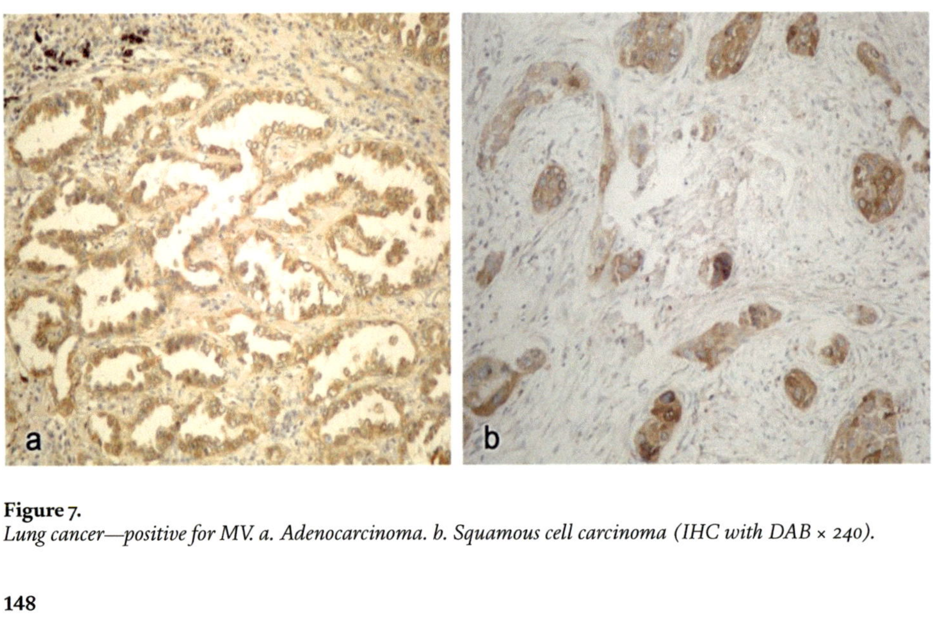

Figure 7.
Lung cancer—positive for MV. a. Adenocarcinoma. b. Squamous cell carcinoma (IHC with DAB × 240).

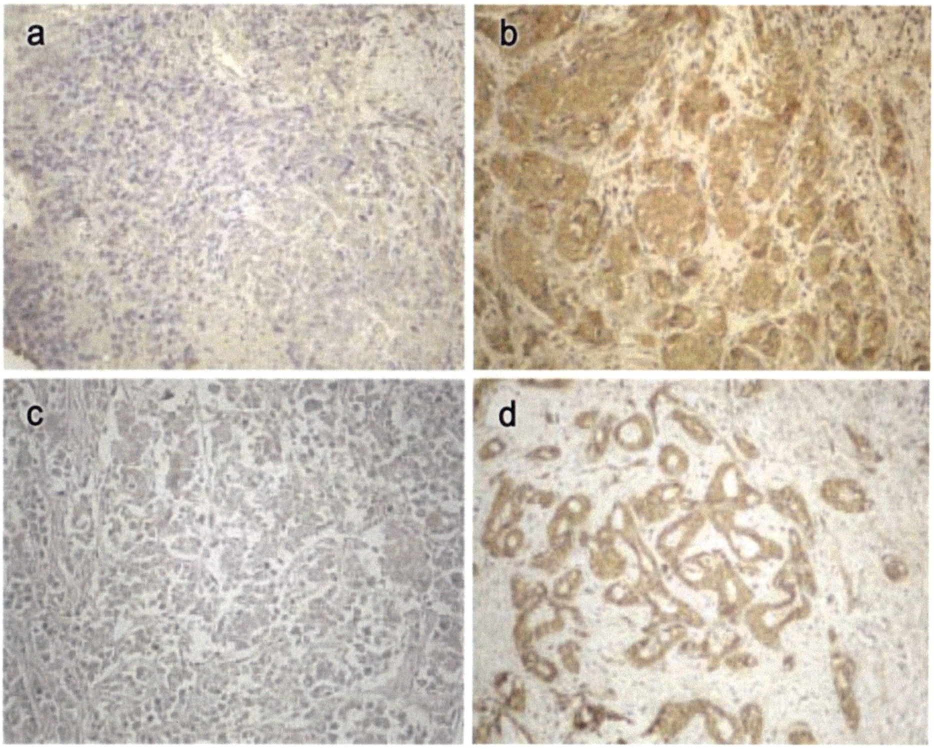

Figure 8.
Breast cancer is positive for measles virus antigens. a and c. Negative controls. b and d. Positive immunostains (immunoperoxidase with DAB × 180).

Variable	Variable distribution	
Demographics		
Age	<50 years	>50 years
Ethnicity	Jewish	Bedouin-Arab
Birth place	Israel/Europe/America	Asia/Africa
Pathology		
Tumor diameter	<10 mm	>10 mm
Axillary LNs	None	Involvement
DCIS component	Yes	No
Grade	Low/intermediate G1–2	High G3
Immunohistochemistry		
ER	Positive	Negative
PR	Positive	Negative
HER2	Positive	Negative
Ki67	Positive	Negative
p53	Positive	Negative
NP-MV	Positive	Negative
HA-MV	Positive	Negative

Table 5.
Distribution of demographics, clinics, pathology, and MV expression in breast cancer patients.

Pathology	Positive (%)	Negative (%)
Adenocarcinoma	11 (84.6%)	2 (15.4%)
Squamous cell carcinoma	3 (100%)	0
Large cell carcinoma	1 (100%)	0
Bronchioloalveolar carcinoma	1 (100%)	0

Table 6.
Western blotting using a phosphoprotein-MV antibody.

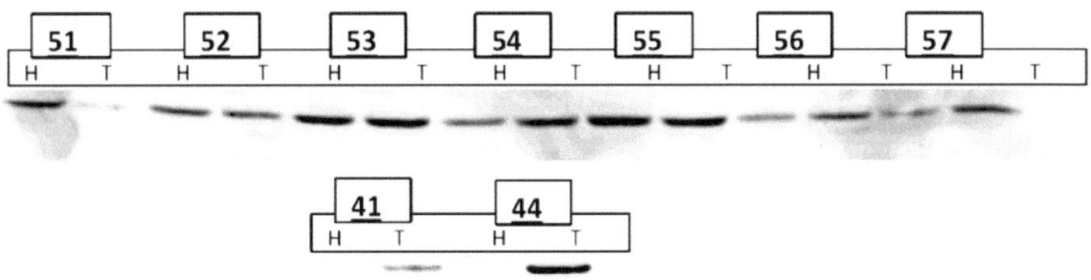

Figure 9.
Western blotting with an antiphosphoprotein-MV antibody on fresh frozen tissues of non-small cell lung cancer. Most cases show positive expression both in tumor tissue (T) and in nonadjacent nonneoplastic lung tissue (H). In a few cases, the MV expression is found in the tumor only.

	Positive staining %			Negative staining %		
Organ	Nucleus	Cytoplasm	Stroma	Nucleus	Cytoplasm	Stroma
Lung	10 (52.6%)	2 (11.1%)	0	9 (47.4%)	16 (88.9%)	18 (100%)
Colon	13 (68.4%)	7 (36.8%)	4 (23.5%)	6 (31.6%)	12 (63.2%)	13 (76.5%)
Stomach	14 (73.7%)	4 (21%)	0	5 (26.3%)	15 (79%)	19 (100%)
Breast	15 (75%)	10 (50%)	2 (10%)	5 (25%)	10 (50%)	18 (90%)

Table 7.
Tissue microarray using a phosphoprotein-MV antibody.

(**Table 6**; **Figure 9**). The second step was to look for the expression of the P-MV in a tissue microarray (one tissue microarray slide). We compared 10 lung cancers, 13 colon cancers, 14 stomach cancers, and 15 breast cancers. Breast cancer expressed the MV antigen in 75% in the nucleus and 50% in the cytoplasm. Stomach cancers expressed the antigen in 73.7% in the nucleus and 21% in the cytoplasm. Colon cancers expressed the MV in 68.4% in the nucleus (**Table 7**). The tissue microarray study had demonstrated a nuclear expression of MV antigens, of which we have not been aware before. This may be due on the one hand to the tiny size of the tissue section. On the other hand, it may be specific to the present anti-P-MV antibody. In any case, various immunostains have shown a marked shuttling of antigens between cytoplasm and nucleus in various tissue sections and with varied antigens [49] (**Table 7**).

Our experience with melanoma and benign melanocytic nevi is shown in **Table 8**. The table shows the expression of several MV antigens and of Pirh2. The expression of NP-MV is the strongest and resembles that of Pirh2. A similar trend, but with a more limited expression, is found in benign melanocytic nevi. It is of note that the expression of the P-protein in melanomas is the mirror image of that of the NP-MV antigen. This was a preliminary exercise and no follow-up is yet

Antigen	Level	Melanoma	Benign nevi	P value
NP-MV	Pos.	46	23	
	Neg.	10	1	0.16
P-protein	Pos.	19	10	
	Neg.	36	12	0.37
HA-MV	Pos.	19	7	
	Neg.	3	1	1.00
Pirh-2	Pos.	44	19	
	Neg.	12	6	0.79

Table 8.
Melanoma and measles virus.

available. The positivity of 23 benign nevi for NP-MV should be investigated to exclude evidence of a pre-malignant condition.

At this stage, we were motivated to determine whether some categories of tumors might be uniformly negative for MV antigens. One limitation is that these tumors were often showed with a restricted sampling. In our original study, we included 25 NHLs by IHC and 7 cases of non-Hodgkin lymphoma by RT-PCR. They were all negative for MV. Only later did we find an interest in ALK-positive anaplastic large cell lymphomas in this regard. In contrast, these lymphomas were predominantly positive for MV. A large scale study of seminomas showed negativity for the MV antigens. Glioblastomas and mesotheliomas were negative for the antigens (Samuel Ariad, personal communication). I later examined small samples of the following tumors which were also negative for the MV antigen: Merkel-cell tumors, hepatocellular carcinoma, malignant mixed mesodermal tumors, and desmoid tumor.

In 2010, we revised and expanded a prior study on the role of apoptosis in CHL [50, 51]. This was undertaken in the light of a consensual point of view: it has been stated that apoptosis in CHL is arrested; this is carried out not only with the help of the NF-κB machinery but also through the expression of EBV-LMP1 that inhibits apoptosis [52–55]. The consensus further determines that this apoptosis hindrance is necessary, since tumor cells in CHL are B cells which cannot express the B-cell receptor (in physiologic conditions, such cells have a strong tendency to die in apoptosis). Thus, apoptosis inhibition is a pre-condition for the survival of H/RS cells [56]. However, in our revision, we found inhibition of H/RS cells apoptosis in 55% of the 217 cases only. Our findings also suggested that NF-κB, specifically the p65 protein, as well as EBV/LMP1 expression did not correlate with apoptosis arrest, in contrast with the consensus view [57]. Of note, it has been shown that although the presence of canonical NF-κB has been considered to be implied, it is the noncanonical NF-κB, which is of predominant relevance in CHL [51]. In the revision we have shown that the most significant association of H/RS cell apoptosis was with p53, the negative expression of which was related with a high apoptotic index (p = 0.001). We looked for a link between positive MV expression and factors related with apoptosis. Associations with apoptotic index less than median (p = 0.005), with MDM2-positive (p = 0.028) and with IκB-positive (p = 0.0001), were displayed. Viruses have a propensity to regulate the apoptotic mechanisms of the infected cell. We have hereby proposed a pathogenic mechanism, involving the MV and that is effective in the modulation of apoptosis, at least in CHL [51].

7. The atypical measles syndrome

In contrast with the classic measles infection, the atypical measles syndrome occurs in older patients, often presenting with a heterogeneous rash, pulmonary infiltrates, hepatic dysfunction, and eosinophilia. The formation of immune complexes has been proposed as responsible for the manifestations of the syndrome [58]. This self-limiting disease, may show, however, long lasting, asymptomatic pulmonary nodules. An immune waning is suspected to occur in this disorder, though such an event has been refuted with measles virus infection at large. Officially, patients with this syndrome have been reported as recently as 2015 [59].

The atypical measles syndrome (AMS) stands out when compared with classic measles for the following reasons.

AMS presents at an older age, often with a high and prolonged fever. A polymorphic rash starts in the hands and feet. In the lungs, this disorder shows nodular infiltrates together with swollen hilar lymph nodes. These changes may regress suddenly. Liver function tests are often abnormal in AMS. Eosinophilia is frequent. This disease entity was first described in 1963, following the vaccination with the formalin inactivated measles virus (FIMV) vaccine. A subsequent exposure to the wild type MV has often been identified. The FIMV vaccine is said to have been withdrawn in 1967, but new cases of AMS were still reported in 2015 [59].

Clinically, the AMS does not resemble the classic MV disease and is usually mild. GPs have difficulties in making the diagnosis in real time. Anti-MV antibody titers are higher than 1:160, which is very unusual for classic measles. In AMS, Koplik spots are frequent and mostly will last 5–7 days, while they last rarely more than 2 days in the classic disease. Photophobia is rarely present in AMS. AMS is probably not contagious [60].

While most cases of AMS in the 1960s were associated with FIMV, the more recent occurrences have been associated with the live attenuated measles vaccine (LAV). Vaccination with FIMV had offered protection for a few months, after which the titers dropped suddenly [61]. We have suggested that this drop of antibody titers is most consistent with a humoral immunity waning. Cases of AMS with prior LAV vaccine have been reported, which are consistent with secondary vaccine failure. Such cases have been suggested to follow a prolonged exposure to an acute measles patient [62].

To confirm the ease by which the diagnosis of AMS is missed, 291 recruits were diagnosed with measles in 1987. They were young adults, with abdominal pain, diarrhea, and vomiting (33%); Koplik spots lasting a mean 7 days; and abnormal liver function tests (86%). The diagnosis of AMS was missed. Retrospectively, this was most certainly the diagnosis, although no anti-MV titers have been reported [63].

In 2015, Levine et al. reported on the status of the measles immunity, 20 years after the two-dose MMR vaccine was introduced. Of the cohort of recruits in 1996, 95.6% had shown positive anti-MV antibodies. In 2007, this positive data had dropped to 85%. Although the authors did not dare to make the statement, this reflected a state of waning immunity, to our opinion [64].

To summarize this issue, we have showed that the AMS differs from typical measles by various features. This is probably a disorder of immunologic nature, involving immune complexes. The AMS is presently rare, but to our opinion, this may be due to a notable under-diagnosis. The association between the AMS pathogenesis and immune waning should be confirmed. It is not excluded that this disorder be related with carcinogenesis as well [65, 66], as it has been proposed that a persistent viral infection is required for virus-associated carcinogenesis [67] and that a waning immunity might lead to a persistent MV infection.

8. Conclusions and prospects

A relationship between MV expression and CHL was provisionally established on IHC [positive with two antigens or more in 82 of 154 CHL patients]; on RT-PCR [positive in 4 of 15 cases for HA-MV RNA; for 2 of 16 NP-MV RNA], and on *in situ* hybridization [for 2 of 7 CHL with HA-MV RNA; in 8 of 21 for NP-MV RNA], as well as with several other malignancies. When focusing on CHL, this association may even be causally linked: apoptosis regulation by the MV may be one of the supportive mechanisms. Our findings are probably sustained by an increasing CHL morbidity related with a progressing occurrence of measles in young adults, in Israel [68], in Quebec [69], and in Connecticut [70], in which frequent outbursts of measles are described.

A clinicopathological correlation, based on the IHC results, was chosen, mainly due to the frequent results as compared with RT-PCR and *in situ* hybridization. In this part of our study, we confirmed an association between CHL and the MV. More females, NS-CHL cases, and more patients in the early stages of their disease were linked to the expression of MV in their tissues. In spite of these variables being, as a rule, correlated with a better prognosis, when they are associated with a positive measles expression, the net effect is a poor prognosis [3].

Regarding the refutation of our findings and conclusions by the German group, this might have been an occasion for further learning. However, the repercussions thereof, on our thesis and our findings, were such that no future was available for us in this domain. As a colleague described it, our position and our theory had been buried. Moreover, I never understood why it was done in that most unpleasant way.

A chapter on the atypical measles syndrome was introduced at the end of the study. This disorder is related with measles and with the MV, but the link has not been clarified completely. Most of the AMS features, clinical, radiological, and biological, differ completely from those of measles. While measles is predominantly an infectious disease, and is highly contagious, AMS is probably not contagious, with its pathogenesis probably based on the formation of immune complexes. One of the highlights of the AMS is an anti-measles antibody titer of 1:160 or higher, much beyond that found in measles. Our interest, at this point, laid in evidence pointing toward immunity waning, as an essential component of AMS. Moreover, in the presence of a sharp drop in the titer, following mainly the FIMV vaccination, as well as occasionally that of the LAV vaccine, the subject might be submitted to the protracted exposition to an acute measles patient. So far, we are not aware of cancer developing in the context of AMS cases, but, since this disorder is often missed, it might be worthwhile looking for cases of cancer within such a context [60].

The prospects and suggestions for proceeding with our research include an epidemiologic study as well as the duplication of our basic investigation, but this once by scientists of good faith. The epidemiologic investigation should have 3 components: the first two, based on our CHL cohort, about half of which show IHC evidence of the MV. Of this population, we will attempt to identify, via the Israeli Ministry of Health Registry, patients who had contracted measles as well as those who had been vaccinated for MV, including vaccination details. The third will deal with AMS, based on the cohorts highlighted by Giladi M et al. [63], and Levine H et al. [64]. Confirmation in the first of the diagnosis of AMS, and research of patients with possibly MV-related tumors and in the second, confirmation of the relevance to immune waning.

Acknowledgements

We thank Kibbutz Sde-Boker for their support.

Conflict of interest

The author declares no conflict of interest.

Notes/thanks/other declarations

Many warm thanks : Samuel Ariad, Martin Sacks, Yonat Shemer-Avni, Yi-Yi Myint, Bracha Rager, Irena Klinkovich, Jacob Gopes, and Eugenia Mejirovski for their valuable contribution.

Author details

Daniel Benharroch
Department of Pathology, Soroka University Medical Center and Faculty of Health Sciences, Ben-Gurion University of the Negev, Beer-Sheva, Israel

*Address all correspondence to: danielbenharroch1@gmail.com

References

[1] Jaffe ES, Stein H, Swerdlow SH. Classic Hodgkin lymphoma. In: Swerdlow SH, Campo E, Harris NL, Jaffe ES, Pileri SA, Stein H, et al., editors. WHO Classification of Tumours of Haematopoietic and Lymphoid Tissues. 4th ed. update. Lyon: IARC; 2017. pp. 435-442

[2] Fend F. Classical Hodgkin's lymphoma and related lesions. In: Jaffe ES, Arber DA, Campo E, Harris NL, Quintanilla-Martinez L, editors. Hematopathology. 2nd ed. Philadelphia: Elsevier; 2017. pp. 525-545

[3] Benharroch D, Shemer-Avni Y, Myint Y-Y, et al. Measles virus: Evidence of an association with Hodgkin's disease. British Journal of Cancer. 2004;**91**:572-579

[4] Benharroch D, Brousset P, Goldstein J, et al. Association of the Epstein-Barr virus with Hodgkin's disease in southern Israel. International Journal of Cancer. 1997;**71**:138-141

[5] Alexander FE, Jarrett RF, Lawrence D, et al. Risk factors for Hodgkin's disease by Epstein-Barr virus (EBV) status: Prior infection by EBV and other agents. British Journal of Cancer. 2000;**82**:1117-1121

[6] Thorley-Lawson DA, Gross A. Mechanisms of disease: Persistence of Epstein-Barr virus and origin of the associated lymphomas. The New England Journal of Medicine. 2004;**350**:1328-1337

[7] Peek RM, Crabtree JE. Helicobacter infection and gastric neoplasia. The Journal of Pathology. 2006;**208**:233-248

[8] Tlsty TD, Coussens LM. Tumor stroma and regulation of cancer development. Annual Review of Pathology. 2006;**1**:119-150

[9] Kundu JK, Surth YJ. Inflammation: Gearing the journey to cancer. Mutation Research. 2008;**659**:15-30

[10] Knecht H, Berger C, Rothenberg S, et al. The role of Epstein-Barr virus in neoplastic transformation. Oncology. 2001;**60**:289-302

[11] Niedobitek G, Meru DHJ. Epstein-Barr virus infection and human malignancies. International Journal of Experimental Pathology. 2001;**82**:149-170

[12] Benharroch D, Shemer-Avni Y, Myint Y-Y, et al. New candidate virus in association with Hodgkin's disease. Leukemia & Lymphoma. 2003;**44**:605-610

[13] Jarrett RF, Armstrong A, Alexander E. Epidemiology of EBV and Hodgkin lymphoma. Annals of Oncology. 1996;**7**(suppl):5-10

[14] Chang KL, Albujar PF, Chen YY, et al. High prevalence of Epstein-Barr virus in Reed-Sternberg cells of Hodgkin disease occurring in Peru. Blood. 1993;**81**:496-501

[15] Gutensohn N, Cole P. Childhood social environment and Hodgkin's disease. The New England Journal of Medicine. 1981;**304**:135-140

[16] Glaser SL. Spacial clustering of Hodgkin's disease in the San Francisco Bay area. American Journal of Epidemiology. 1990;**132**(Suppl):s167-s177

[17] Westergaard T, Melbye M, Pedersen JB, et al. Birth order, sibship size and the risk of Hodgki's disease in children and young adults: A population based study of 31 million person-years. International Journal of Cancer. 1997;**72**:977-981

[18] Sleckman BG, Mauch PM, Ambinder RF, et al. Epstein-Barr virus

in Hodgkin's disease: Correlation of risk factors and disease characteristics with molecular evidence of viral infection. Cancer Epidemiology, Biomarkers & Prevention. 1998;**7**:1117-1121

[19] Glaser SL, Clark CA, Nugent RA, et al. Social class and risk of Hodgkin's disease in young adult women in 1988-94. International Journal of Cancer. 2002;**98**:110-117

[20] Torreli G, Marasca R, Lupi M, et al. Human herpesvirus-6 in human lymphomas: Identification of specific sequences in Hodgkin's lymphoma by polymerase chain reaction. Blood. 1991;**77**:2251-2258

[21] Armstrong AA, Shield L, Gallagher A, et al. Lack of involvement of known oncogenic DNA viruses in Epstein-Barr negative Hodgkin's disease. British Journal of Cancer. 1998;**77**:1045-1047

[22] Berneman ZN, Torreli G, Luppi M, et al. Absence of a directly causative role for herpesvirus-7 in human lymphoma and a review of human herpesvirus-6 in human malignancy. Annals of Hematology. 1998;**77**:275-278

[23] Cozen W, Masood R, Mack T, et al. Seroprevalence of Kaposi's sarcoma-associated herpesvirus antibody in young adult Hodgkin's disease. Blood. 1998;**91**:724

[24] Jarret RF, MacKenzie J. Epstein-Barr virus and other candidate viruses in the pathogenesis of Hodgkin's disease. Seminars in Hematology. 1999;**36**:260-269

[25] Schmidt CA, Oettle H, Peng R, et al. Presence of β- and γ-herpes virus DNA in Hodgkin's disease. Leukemia. 2000;**24**:865-870

[26] Gallager A, Perry J, Shield L, et al. Viruses and Hodgkin's disease: No evidence of novel herpesvirus in non-EBV-associated lesions. International Journal of Cancer. 2002;**101**:259-264

[27] Gopas J, Shemer-Avni Y, Levy A, et al. Measles virus expression in Hodgkin's lymphoma. Proceedings of the American Association for Cancer Research. 2001;**42**:111 (Abstract)

[28] Kamel OW, Le Brun DP, Berry GJ, et al. Warthin-Finkeldey polykaryotes demonstrate a T-cell immunophenotype. American Journal of Clinical Pathology. 1992;**97**:179-183

[29] Griffin DE, Pan CH. Measles virus. In: Griffin DE, Oldstone MBA, editors. Measles Pathogenesis and Control. Berlin: Springer; 2009

[30] Birrer MJ, Bloom BR, Udem R. Characterization of measles polypeptides by monoclonal antibodies. Virology. 1981;**108**:381-390

[31] Schneider-Schaulies S, Lieber UG, Segev Y, et al. Antibody-dependent transcriptional regulation of measles virus in persistently infected neural cells. Journal of Virology. 1992;**66**:5534-5541

[32] Ogata A, Czub S, Ogata S, et al. Absence of measles virus receptor (CD46) in lesions of subacute sclerosis panencephalitis brains. Acta Neuropathologica. 1997;**94**:444-449

[33] Dickinson HO, Tyari TA, Parker L. Childhood solid tumors in relation to infections in the community in Cumbria during pregnancy and around the time of birth. British Journal of Cancer. 2002;**87**: 746-750

[34] Tyari TA, Dickinson HO, Parker L. Childhood cancer in relation with infections in the community during pregnancy and around the time of birth. International Journal of Cancer. 2003;**104**:772-777

[35] Zygiert Z. Hodgkin's disease: Remission after measles. Lancet. 1971;**1**(7699):593

[36] Mota HC. Infantile Hodgkin's disease: Remission after measles. British Medical Journal. 1973;**2**:241

[37] Zwitter M. Hodgkin's disease: Therapeutic role of measles vaccine. American Journal of Medicine. 1984;**77**:A49, A52, A64

[38] Schattner A. Therapeutic role of measles vaccine in Hodgkin's disease. Lancet. 1984;**1**(8469):171

[39] Cozen W, Hamilton AS, Zaho P, et al. A protective role for early oral exposures in the etiology of young adult Hodgkin's lymphoma. Blood. 2009;**114**:4014-4020

[40] Maggio E, Benharroch D, Gopas J, et al. Absence of measles virus genome and transcripts in Hodgkin/Reed-Sternberg cells of a cohort of Hodgkin lymphoma patients. International Journal of Cancer. 2007;**121**:448-453

[41] Wilson KS, Freeland JML, Gallagher A, et al. Measles virus and classical Hodgkin lymphoma: No evidence for a direct association. International Journal of Cancer. 2007;**121**:242-247

[42] Karlin D, Belshaw R. Detecting remote sequence homology in disorsered proteins: Discovery of conserved motifs in the N-termini of Mononrgavirales phosphoproteins. PLoS One. 2012;7:e31719

[43] Kruzniar A, van Ham RC, Pongor S, et al. The quest for orthologs: Finding the corresponding gene across genomes. Trends in Genetics. 2008;**24**:539-551

[44] Benharroch D, Klinkovich I, Piura B, et al. Evidence of measles virus antigens and RNA in endometrial cancer. European Journal of Obstetrics, Gynecology, and Reproductive Biology. 2009;**147**:206-209

[45] Duan W, Gao L, Druhon LJ, et al. Expression of Pirh2, a newly identified ubiquitin protein ligase in lung cancer. Journal of the National Cancer Institute. 2004;**96**:1718-1721

[46] Sion-Vardy N, Lazarev I, Delgado B, et al. Measles virus: Evidence for association with lung cancer. Experimental Lung Research. 2009;**35**:701-712

[47] Ariad S, Milk N, Bolotin A, et al. Measles virus antigens in breast cancer. Anticancer Research. 2011;**31**:913-920

[48] Chen M, Cortay J-C, Logan IR, et al. Inhibition of ubiquitination and stabilisation of human ubiquitin E3 ligase Pirh2 by measles virus phosphoprotein. Journal of Virology. 2005;**79**:11824-11836

[49] Nihie T, Nagata K, Takeuchi K. The C protein of wild-type measles virus has the ability to shuttle between the nucleus and the cytoplasm. Microbes and Infection. 2007;**9**:344-354

[50] Benharroch D, Levy A, Prinsloo I, et al. Apoptotic index as a prognostic factor in Hodgkin's disease. Leukemia & Lymphoma. 1999;**33**:351-359

[51] Benharroch D, Einav I, Feldman A, et al. Apoptosis of Hodgkin-Reed-Sternberg cells in classical Hodgkin lymphoma revisited. Acta Pathologica, Microbiologica, et Immunologica Scandinavica. 2010;**118**:339-345

[52] Marafioti T, Hummel M, Foss HD, et al. Hodgkin and reed-Sternberg cells represent an expansion of a single clone originating from a germinal center B-cell with functional Ig gene rearrangement but defective Ig transcription. Blood. 2000;**95**:1443-1450

[53] Kuppers R, Rajewsky K. The origin of Hodgkin-Reed-Sternberg cells in Hodgkin's disease. Annual Review of Immunology. 1998;**16**:471-493

[54] Kuppers R, Hansmann ML, Rajewsky K, et al. Clonality and germinal center derivation of Hodgkin/Reed-Sternberg cells in Hodgkin's disease. Annals of Oncology. 1998;**9**(suppl 5):s17-s20

[55] Kuppers R. Molecular biology of Hodgkin's lymphoma. Advances in Cancer Research. 2002;**84**:277-312

[56] Bargou RC, Emmerich F, Krappmann D, et al. Constitutive nuclear factor-κB, RelA activation is required for proliferation and survival of Hodgkin's disease tumor cells. The Journal of Clinical Investigation. 1997;**100**:2961-2969

[57] Izban KF, Ergin M, Huang Q, et al. Characterization of NF-κB expression in Hodgkin's disease. Modern Pathology. 2001;**14**:297-310

[58] Griffin DE, Pan CH. Inactivated vaccines. In: Griffin DE, Oldstone MBA, editors. Measles Pathogenesis and Control. Berlin: Springer; 2009. pp. 194-195

[59] Melenotte C, Cassir N, Tessonier L, et al. Atypical measles syndrome in adults: Still around. BMJ Case Reports. 2015:**2015**

[60] Benharroch D. Atypical measles syndrome—A brief review. Annals of Clinical Cytology and Pathology. 2016;**2**:1039-1041

[61] Rauh LW, Schmidt R. Measles immunization with killed virus vaccine. Serum antibody titers and experience with exposure to measles epidemic. American Journal of Diseases of Children. 1965;**109**:232-237

[62] Hickman CJ, Hyde TB, Sowers SB, et al. Laboratory characterization of measles virus infection in previously vaccinated and unvaccinated individuals. Journal of Infectious Diseases. 2011;**204**:s549-s558

[63] Giladi M, Schulman A, Kedem R, et al. Measles in adults: A prospective study of 291 consecutive cases. British Medical Journal. 1987;**295**:1314

[64] Levine H, Zarka S, Ankol OE, et al. Seroprevalence of measles, mumps and rubella among young adults, after 20 years of universal 2-dose MMR vaccination in Israel. Human Vaccines & Immunotherapeutics. 2015;**11**:1400-1405

[65] Wood DL, Brunell PA. Measles control in the United States: Problems of the past and challenges for the future. Clinical Microbiology Reviews. 1995;**8**:260-267

[66] Kontio M, Jokinen S, Paunio M, et al. Waning antibody levels and avidity: Implications for the MMR vaccine-induced protection. The Journal of Infectious Diseases. 2012;**206**:1542-1548

[67] Dziurzyski K, Chang SM, Heimberger AB, et al. Consensus on the role of human cytomegalovirus in glioblastoma. Neuro-Oncology. 2012;**14**:246-255

[68] Ariad S, Lipshitz I, Benharroch D, et al. A sharp rise in the incidence of Hodgkin's lymphoma in young adults in Israel. The Israel Medical Association Journal. 2009;**11**:453-455

[69] Liu S, Semensiw R, Waters C, et al. Time trends and sex patterns in Hodgkin's disease in Canada, 1970-1995. Canadian Journal of Public Health. 2000;**91**:188-192

[70] Chen YT, Zheng T, Chou MC, et al. The increase in Hodgkin's disease incidence among young adults. Experience in Connecticut, 1935-1992. Cancer. 1997;**79**:2209-2218